# F CANC___, MIRACLE CURE FOR CANCER

The Story Of A Writer Who Used To Be A Pharmaceutical Chemical Researcher Has Cured Himself And Helped His Friend Cure Cancer

DONG LA

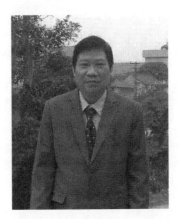

## ĐÔNG LA - NGUYỄN HUY HÙNG

(Writer and pharmaceutical chemical researcher)

*Prize A of science and technology Competition in HCM city 1993.
*Annual award of the Union of Vietnam Arts and Literature Association 2013.

*Born June 30, 1955, in Hai Duong Province, Viet Nam, is a writer who used to be a pharmaco-chemical researcher.

*1976-1981: studied Chemical Faculty of University of Ho Chi Minh City. 1981-1990: worked in the Institute of Pharmaceutical Industry under the Ministry of Health of Vietnam.

*1990-1995: worked in the Agricultural Chemical Research Center of Vietnam Pesticides Company.

# Table of Contents

# INTRODUCTION

Today, people are no stranger to vegetarian diets for better health. It stems from the application of the "Macrobiotic" diet, which is based on George Oshawa's yin-yang balance concept. This principle has the mystery color of eastern philosophy, but from the point of view of modern science, it is not clear.

So in fact, there are many people who have been healed by this vegetarian diet, but modern medicine still does not believe it. So it has not been thoroughly researched, and it's still too far to be applied even if the hospitals have failed to treat cancer for these patients.

And more positive, to cure cancer, some people practice "hunger strike" in the selected time period with the hope that this helps by cutting nutrient supply to the tumor and kill it.

Perhaps, this is because people do not understand the deep meaning of those two methods. A doctor said: *"Many cancer patients think that they do not eat to heal because they are afraid that cancer cells will develop if they eat a lot".*

*"This is a very wrong concept. More patients die as a result of poor diet regime than from cancer."*

Another doctor said:

*"If the patients don't eat or drink, their energy gets depleted. They will be too weak and unhealthy to reduce the risk of recurrence of cancer, prevents metastases."*

But the fact is that vegetarians are not only healthy, but are also cured of many diseases, including cancer. This is simply because eating a plant food source may lack some essential amino acids, but if you eat a variety of foods, you get all you need.

People who try "hunger-strike" as a solution to cancer can die of hunger before dying of cancer?

You need to understand, that "hunger-strike" here is under control. The time sufficient for fasting for each person depends on the individual's body weight and of course the amount of fat stored in the body. So, you should practice "hunger strike" in a suitable time, not "hunger-strike" to die!

There are many ways of explaining the mechanism of cancer treatment by vegetarian, I personally see the tumor as a plant sprout, it grows stronger than the body, so it needs nutrition many times than the body's normal requirements. It's the main source of nutrient is animal protein, so cut off this nutrient supply from your diet, it will die. Excess intake of animal protein only serves to "fatten" the tumor.

The method drawn from using food to fight cancer is thought to be very simple, but difficult to implement.

In order to change from a normal diet to a vegetarian diet, we must overcome habits and appetites. But again, failing to eat only makes us very hungry. For me, the author of this book, when I discovered that my mole was at risk for skin cancer, I had a "hunger strike," only drinking coconut water for more than ten days, and finally the miracle, that risk mole has fallen out. It feels terrible when suffering from hunger, but you eventually overcome it. But between hunger and death, one must make a choice, and I chose hunger.

From that fact base, I studied the causes of cancer and how to treat it with a diet based on physiology and biochemistry of the body. From the nutritional needs of the body, the process of metabolism and how it creates energy for the body to function, the protein synthesis in the cell (for cell regeneration maintaining the body functionality), to recognize the harmful health factors. In addition to this, I also learned the causes of cancer as sabotage of free radicals and excess nutrients. This is how I found the way to stop. In it, I found that deepest secrete of the vegetarian diet to cured cancer is that it offers dietary intake in which the essential amino acids does not exceed the needs of the body requirement.

Only shortage of one essential amino acid, the whole protein chain will not be formed during the synthesis of the cell, the tumor cannot grow, it will die, and finally, the patient is the winner!

*Los Angeles*

*2- 9- 2017*

*ĐÔNG LA*

# PART I: WIN THE FIGHT AGAINST CANCER

## The story of a writer who used to be pharmaceutical chemical researcher, himself and help his friend cure cancer

I studied Chemical Faculty of University of Ho Chi Minh City. In year-ends, I was also selected for the training of University lecturer and researchers at research institutes.

Study finished, I applied to teach at a university and was accepted, but I was also invited to work at a pharmacy research institute by an officer of the institute. Being the Institute of Pharmaceutical Industry under the Ministry of Health of Vietnam, I dropped out teaching at the University and opted to work in this research institute.

In the research institute, the first thing I work focused on was to work a team that extracts active ingredient is Berberine of "vàng đắng" tree. Its scientific name is Coscinium usitatum, which grows in the forest of Vietnam. Berberine is an alkaloid used to treat diarrhea, dysentery, intestinal inflammation, jaundice, fever, malaria, poor digestion, and eye pain.

Then I worked on many other projects, but the most memorable was being assigned to lead a research team to extract Vinblastine substance from "Dừa cạn" tree, whose scientific name is Catharanthus roseus or Vinca rose. This plant grows wild and is grown as an ornamental plant. Vinblastin is used to treat leukemia (the cancer of white blood cells).

The content of vinblastine in Vinca rose is very low, only about 1 in 10,000. Only 1 kg of vinblastine can be extracted from 10 tons of Vinca rose. So, the work was very difficult. We extracted with ethanol (Ethanol, $C_2H_5OH$), concentrated, refined to obtain the total alkaloid. Next we poured the total alkaloid solution flowing through the chromatography columns; the active ingredients gradually gets separated. We then took parts containing Vinblastine and allowed it to concentrate and crystallize into the crystal of Vinblastine. We obtained Vinblastine from this.

Vinblastine is valued at very high price. We hear people say that it costs millions of dollars per kilogram. In the laboratory scale, we did a few grams.

I was very happy, prepared to study on a larger scale. But then, a surprise happened. The team leader of research (me) was replaced simply because the new leader of the research institute was promoted. The incoming boss who happened to be a woman did not like me at all. The year was 1989. I was sad but not surprised because after nearly ten years in the research institute, I knew that there was a deep division among the group of leaders of the institute. Different factions fought each other for the position of Directorship of the research institute. Short story, the first literary work of my writing life is "The story of two people" which talks about that fight, and that is the main reason the leader of the institute did not want me to continue working in the research institute. I was very sad to have to suddenly drop the project that was not yet completed. It felt as though a baby was removed from his mom. But after I left, the fight continued, my research institute finally broke down, and of course, my anti-cancer research work was never completed.

Then I applied for a job at the Agricultural Chemical Research Center of Vietnam Pesticides Company. Here I was again assigned to lead a team and continuing to research and to produce a pest control product that preserves postharvest agricultural products. This project had lasted for more than 20 years but had never been completed because the Active ingredient of that product causes fire and explosions. After three years, I finished that work. An International Workshop on Reducing Postharvest Loss tested my product with 18 participating countries (hosted by ACCT and Bordeaux) in Binh Tay rice warehouse and it was evaluated and found to be equivalent to the German product. A member of the French delegation asked to buy our products for use in France. Then my research work was sent to the contest in "Creative Science and Technology" of Ho Chi Minh City 1993 and I was awarded A which was the highest award.

Obviously, I have the ability to do scientific research, but I do not know my sad story when working in that research institute is because of the social reality or because of my destiny.

I have applied for no longer work at state agency, I chose to work from home. I have created some nutrition products for the plant, set up production and businesses to create wealth for my wife and children. And I have a mission, I have to write. At first, I wrote poetry, then wrote short stories, and then literary criticism. Finally, I am an experienced and knowledgeable writer, the front of the vibrant life, there is a lot of good and evil is not clear. The society has many weaknesses and wrongs. So, I wrote a lot to discuss about politics, was admitted as a member of the Vietnam Writers Association.

As usual, I lost a lot, so perhaps, I should go "fight" against the state of Vietnam like many people on behalf of "dissent" in Vietnam. But I only wrote critiques, pointing out the mistakes and weaknesses of Vietnamese society but with constructive attitude. I expected Vietnam to stabilize and develop. I also opposed those who take advantage of the freedom of speech, take advantage of the failures of the Vietnamese society, exaggerate and distort to fight the regime, destabilize for the Vietnamese society and the peaceful life its citizens.

Even with this, I still remain a science researcher, I always enjoy reading, learning, updating achievements in many fields of science, and when I get older, I pay close attention to the research results related to health care, especially healthy diet that can treat diseases including cancer.

More than a dozen years ago, when my acquaintance had cancer, I studied cancer treatment by Japanese vegetarian diet. The method has many mystical complex arguments of the East, but as the researcher; I understood that the deepest nature of the problem is to cut off the essential amino acid supply to the tumor. The animal protein contains too much essential amino acids, far much more than the body requires. The excess amino acids only goes to feed and fatten the tumor.

If only an essential amino acids is lacking, the cell will not have a "brick" attached to the amino acid chain that makes up the complete protein for the tumor growth, and it will starve and die. But my acquaintances don't understand this fact, they are not willing to become a vegetarian. To make it worse, their meal plans contains too much meat. This may be the reason they end up dead in a matter of time.

A few years ago, I saw the mole under my left eye, it was growing fast and itches too! I was afraid it can turn into melanoma. No need to go to the clinic, my plan was to treat myself with meals. I neither ate animal meat or anything else, I only took coconut juice. To make this change was difficult, but again, I knew very well what the fight was about. It was cancer, and cancer is synonymous with death as we know it. So, the choice was not as difficult. Finally, the result is wonderful, after about 10 days only drinking coconut juice, the mole gradually shed and fall off! I know that it has turned into melanoma because just like that, it was affected by eating, many other normal moles on my body are still intact.

A few months ago, before going to the US, a friend of mine made an appointment with me after he had surgery to remove the liver cancer. We met and I advised him to consider the Japanese vegetarian diet. I am a writer so I also updated my readers through blog posts. I taught them how to apply this amazing Japanese vegetarian diet. With my blogs up, sometimes thousands of people were reading my posts all at the same time.

## Số lượt xem theo quốc gia

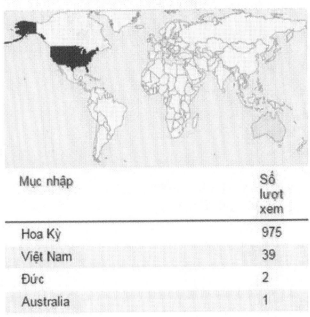

| Mục nhập | Số lượt xem |
|---|---|
| Hoa Kỳ | 975 |
| Việt Nam | 39 |
| Đức | 2 |
| Australia | 1 |

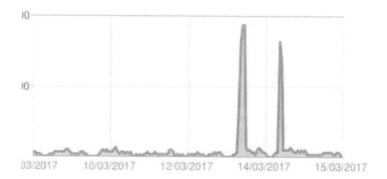

But sadly, one day, I saw my wrist, the part I wear the watch had a purple-black spot. Again melanoma! Even though I once successfully treated myself with melanoma, I was still very worried. It seems that God has challenged me; I have to do it again, as people used to say, "Words must have books, advice must have evidence". When I advise my friends, I must do the same.

The details of that story and what its outcome will look like is the content of this book.

This is a true story of real people. The author hopes people find, read and applies it when needed. Only with determination and understanding, not the money, the patient can still when the fight against cancer. Unlike most other diseases, it is often discovered late. To make it worse, the modern medicine does little to help people prevent it.

*Los Angeles*

*2-9-2017*

*ĐÔNG LA*

## Visit my friend who has liver cancer

Before the Lunar New Year, I got a phone call:

*"Mr. Hung (my real name), after the Lunar New Year, I went to Cho Ray Hospital for re-examination, we will meet each other! I was very sick so we could not talk at length, we arrived to catch up and talk later."*

Although my friend did not insist on details, I still felt very bad. Later on February 16 (solar calendar), we met again, he told me that he had to come to the hospital for tests because he had a surgery for liver cancer!

******

Again Cho Ray Hospital, again cancer! Cho Ray Hospital has so many unforgettable things in my life.

In 1989, the great poet Che Lan Vien in Vietnam, whom I considered as my father, had been examined by the doctor and discovered to have lung cancer. The doctor recommended surgery for him at the Cho Ray hospital. That day, I witnessed the moment the nurse pushed the stretcher out of the operating room. His face was swollen. He had a lung operation so it was very hard to breathe. His body was covered with a white cloth. After the operation, he recovered really fast, and in a matter of time, he appeared normal, as though nothing happened. When we thought everything was well, metastasis was developing from inside. The Cancer cells run to the brain creating a tumor. He started losing consciousness. Then boom! Just like that, he was gone forever!

The second story is again that of a close friend of mine. This man used to live in my village. His wife was diagnosed with brain tumor and the doctors at Cho Ray Hospital operated her. I still remember that day vividly. I also saw people push the stretcher from the operating room to her room, in the same room there was a girl who had been operated earlier, it seems the anesthetic was gone, she was moaning pain! After that, she recovered quickly. Just like Che Lan Vien, she soon suffered from a metastatic tumor, lost consciousness and she finally died.

Now my friend also has liver cancer. Unfortunately for most Vietnamese, when one is diagnosed with cancer, it was always at the late stage. It was more like a death sentence to them. Just like singer Tran Lap recently singing on television, then came singer Minh Thuan also fun in the "familiar faces" program, both died because of cancer. When it comes to cancer treatment, the surgeons often opt for the surgical procedure to remove the tumor. This is followed by series of chemotherapy and radiotherapy. The success rate of surgical procedure in the remove of the tumor can only be high if the disease was detected early and the tumors are small. The doctors are able to remove all tumors, no cancer cells remain, and the patient will be cured. But if the disease is late, the tumor has grown, despite the surgery, the remaining cancer cells will still spread to other parts of the body, forming new tumors. So, after surgery, doctors often perform chemotherapy and radiation. But not only chemotherapy kills cancer cells but also destroys healthy cells in the bone marrow, stomach and intestines, and can cause damage to organs like the liver, kidneys, heart, and lungs.

The radiation in the process of destroying cancer cells can also damage healthy cells and organs. Chemotherapy and radiation usually reduce the size of the tumor at its initial stages. The long-term use will not destroy the tumor anymore, causing the immune system to be damaged or destroyed, so the body will not be able to withstand infections and complications. Chemotherapy and radiation can also cause cancer cells to mutate and become resistant and difficult to destroy. So when the cancer is discovered late, the tumor has grown up, it's like boxer still "knock out" modern medicine.

When Poet Che Lan Vien was sick, I was the head of the project to extract the anti-cancer substance Vinblastine from the Vinca rose tree. I know that cancer can only be treated at an early stage, Vinblastine is often used for the treatment of blood cancer, I knew it was useless, but I still took a bottle of medicine for writer Vu Thi Thuong, his wife, give him drink, and true it was useless.

Next, this man who came from my village found himself in the same predicament. His wife was diagnosed with brain cancer. I went to the bookstore to find some books that could assist me in the research work. I noticed the book "Methods of eating to prevent cancer" of the Japanese

15

edited by Pham Thi Ngoc Tram. I bought several of these books to keep should any of my acquaintances need one for their own use. In addition to home reading, I used to be a research fellow at the Institute of Pharmaceutical Industry of the Ministry of Health.

I found that the treatment of cancer of the Japanese by diet is true. Then learnt more about physiology, biochemistry, metabolism in the human body. I found that curing cancer by eating also have a scientific basis. That method is simple, just a fully vegetarian diet! If combined "hunger-strike" with the appropriate duration, the method is more effective.

I was overjoyed to give this man from my village the book. Unfortunately, the couple (the man and his wife) were unable to understand the deeper meaning of this book. Their area of specialization was the social field, and nothing much to say about medicine. So he still allows his wife to eat meat-rich meals that is contrary to the healing base of the book. I can't stop him because the couple loves each other and denying his wife to do what she wants goes against their love. As a result, she died. Then comes the story of my wife. Her uncle is a priest and the head of the church of Chi Hoa. He was also diagnosed with liver cancer, after years of B virus infection. I also gave him that book on cancer treatment by that vegetarian diet and show off teaching science for a preacher. He listened to me, vegetarian for a while, very happy to be effective. When he went to see the doctor, he was informed that his liver enzymes decreased. But some Sueur because too loves their priest, went to buy some "ac" chicken to cook with "Bac" drug for their father to eat. "The enthusiasm with the ignorance is destructive"; love each other without understanding might only lead to death. In this case, the "ac" chicken is literally evil, it does not foster patients, and it nourishes the tumor. Having eaten, my wife's uncle was taken to the emergency hospital and he was dead a few days later.

******

Knowing my friend had cancer, I went looking for the book on cancer prevention by a vegetarian diet. I photocopied the book and took one copy to my friend.

Afternoon 16-2, my friend called:

*"Mr. Hung, I'm done with the examination. Please come to Cho Ray Hospital. When you arrive, give me a call, I will come out".*

I went to the hospital, after a few years we met again, I saw my friend changed so much, his face looked pale and gray. His hair and beard were white, but he was still fun, no pessimism.

I drove him to a cafe nearby and said:

*"Now you say you are focused on your "strategy" treatment. If I see you aren't right, I will suggest for you."*

*"I'm generally vegetarian and meditating."*

*"That is the right direction, but what really matters is whether you can maintain it or not. You have to win yourself, you must beat the poor eating habits, and beat the greediness. Talking is easy but doing is very difficult. In short, you have to completely eat vegetarian food."*

Last "TET", had full of fish and meat but the whole month I only ate vegetables, tubers, fruits, and drunk some milk to get protein.

At this point, I gave him the book and said:

*"Drinking milk is wrong, I am giving you this book to read. First, read the story of the doctor in the United States that had cancer, when he was pushed to the end of the road, he turned to the vegetarian Japanese style to treat the disease. But he kept strict discipline, still going to work, meetings, partying, but he was always carrying a box of vegetarian rice to eat alone. There are many ways of explaining the mechanism of cancer treatment by vegetarian, I personally see this, the tumor is like a plant sprout, it grows stronger than the body, so it needs more nutrition, and its main nutrient is animal protein. If you cut off the source of the nutrient supply to it, it dies. This explained the cases of cancer patients going on "hunger-strike", and the tumor dies before the body. There was a woman who had a tumor in her nostril, she tried hunger strike and finally saw it fall out. But people who choose "hunger-strike" must have a very strong will if they are to succeed."*

*"So, I will also eliminate the milk I bought into the hospital. It was sold to parents to drink and I had bought some for the family use back at home."*

Finished speaking, he took the cigarettes in his bag to invite me, I shook my head, and he lit a cigarette to smoke and asked:

*"Have you given up on smoking? I also gave up but sometimes I still smoke."*

*"So you are wrong, discipline is not strict, you should remember that you are facing possible death, you can die just like a house mouse, or just like cockroaches die. I am a writer, have to illustrate using photos to impress you. Now you have to quit right away. It is not just about lung cancer, when smoking, the toxins and other free radicals infiltrate the blood. In case of normal people, they may not be affected as much, but with you, the cells have been and are still sprouting to form cancer, they only need a slight stimulation and they will grow."*

*"So I will also quit smoking completely!"*

\*\*\*\*\*\*

I thought I told everything I needed to say to a friend who was carrying a serious illness, so I left. But I knew it was still very difficult, even myself, I'm highly knowledgeable, but I don't easily escape the dangerous habits. Whether it is the eating habit, the living habit or even those habits that are harmful to health, it is all difficult.

Perhaps, with a polite man, people often talk fun, and success stories. When they inadvertently talk about the illness of others they have to apologize. But this is not a polite story; it's a story of life and death. I want to write for my friend so that he can understand the problem better and to have more will and more confidence in understanding the scientific basis, as well as practicality overcome the dangerous disease.

I don't understand why I had to put so much effort on such overly high scientific theories as; General Theory of Relativity, Quantum Mechanics, and Unified field theory to make a dialogue with people who do not understand. The reason as to why I do not write to share my insights about things closer and important to everyone is that eating is not just to sustain life but also to protect the health and treat diseases.

# The scientific basis of the diet to fight cancer

Today I am going to write in detail about vegetarianism against cancer. I write broadly on the scientific and practical basis of vegetarianism against cancer.

\*\*\*\*\*\*

Before I write, I will share an interesting story about the friend who had liver cancer. We met after a while when he had shared his Facebook information probably to certify if the words I had told him were true.

He said that he had a friend had Lung cancer since he had a malignant lump as big as a teacup in his lungs. Sadly, the doctor told him to go home and wait to die. The tumor could not be cut because it was close to the aorta. Back at home, he started his own therapy through avoiding sugar, meat, fish, rice and just drinking a mixture water of vegetables, carrots, radishes, beetroot, oranges, and apples. After three months, the tumor decreased its size a lot and after nine months the cancerous tumor completely disappeared. Now he is healthy, working and eating normally. Have cancer just like him, chemical therapy was used on four people who had cancer and they were dead.

\*\*\*\*\*\*

Each body is maintained alive by physiological and biochemical processes. There are normalized definitions in the syllabus but I still want to redefine in a neat way. "Physiology is all the activities of the organs of the body, while biochemistry is the chemical nature of those physiological activities. The end of these activities is the metabolism of chemicals to maintain the body structure, maintain the body's functional activities and ultimately generate energy to provide for all those activities of the body."

Metabolism of substances to sustain life at the same time also has side effects and is the cause of illnesses, including cancer.

We all know that in addition to the small amounts of minerals and vitamins, the human body needs mainly water, oxygen and a component that not only maintains life, but also makes people happy. That is food. Foods have three main groups: Lipids, Carbohydrates, and Proteins.

In a textbook, an Associate Professor Ph.D. at Hanoi Medical University wrote:

"Proteins has a major role to play in the composition of all the cells, shaping the body."

It is in the muscle, in the cell nucleus (the structure of DNA and RNA), in plasma (albumin, globulin, and fibrinogen). Proteins are also a major component of antibodies and enzymes in the body. Proteins have a decisive role in genetics. The genes of each individual are located on the DNA molecule that determines the genetic characteristics of the individual and the species.

The Proteins of the human body is made up of 20 different amino acids, including 10 amino acids that the body does not synthesize or synthesize only a small amount compared to the needs of the body, so must be taken from the outside. They are called essential amino acids, including Threonine, methionine, valine, leucine, isoleucine, lysine, arginine, phenylalanine, tryptophan, and histidine.

The Proteins of each animal in the daily diet has a different amino acid ratio and differs from that of humans so it is important to have to eat a variety of Proteins of different animals such as fish, poultry, pork, meat cow ... In milk, vegetables and rice also have a certain ratio of Proteins but low Proteins content, so the number of Proteins provided is still mostly from animals. "

The above is not a personal opinion but the theory of modern medicine. Thus, the problem with vegetarians is that they eat vegetable protein instead of animal protein which can't cure cancer but also against modern Medical. However, there are many people cured of cancer by the vegetarian diet which modern medicine still does not believe, so it is not studied thoroughly and still too far to be able to be applied. In addition, there are rare cases people cured of cancer by strange treatments and other mysterious methods, which modern medicine still considers it as myths and superstitions.

I'm close to Vu This Hoa, a patient with uterine cancer; the hospital took her to her home waiting to die. She had been treated from a "Man" man over 90 years old, by his herbal remedies and "holy water". She died clinically until a few days before her tumor had broken. Then she recovered and both she and her family were surprised that she gradually found herself with strange abilities, including seeing the soul of the dead and she was also able to cure some cancer patients. The first patient is her ex-husband, Mr. Suu, who had stomach cancer; the hospital also took him to his home waiting to die. And the photo below is a woman whose name is Ms. Minh lives in Vung Tau city. She was kneeling in front of Ms. Vu Thi Hoa. Personally, I have met her several times. She was kneeling in front of Vu Thi Hoa because she considered Ms. Hoa as the Bodhisattva who saved her life from bladder cancer.

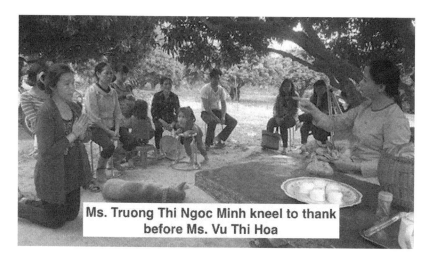

Ms. Truong Thi Ngoc Minh kneel to thank before Ms. Vu Thi Hoa

This is a fact; which reality is not only the mother of medicine but also the father of science. The reality of life always poses problems such as math tests that do not yet have answers, forcing science to answer, thus promoting the development of science.

Vegetarians should know what to eat and how to eat enough for the demand of the body is another subject will be discussed later. This article mainly discusses the harmful effects of eating animal meat for patients who have cancer. So, the patient should be a vegetarian, using vegetable protein instead of animal protein.

Eating meat, especially red meat, the metabolism of substances in the body can cause the following three major effects:

- Create an acid environment in the body.

- Ion Fe excess causing harm.

- Creates free radicals.

*****

The ancients taught us, *"know the enemy, know ourselves, fight hundred battle, win hundred,"* so we need to know the enemy of health so that we can prevent and eliminate them.

## 1- Acidic environment:

For the body to function, nutrients such as proteins, Carbohydrates, and lipid will need to be oxidized, releasing a lot of energy, some of it radiating in the form of heat, in part create substance adenosine triphosphate (ATP). It is a repository because the body only uses energy in the form of ATP:

# Adenosine triphosphat

Continuous energy is generated and circulated within the cell for use through the transformation of ATP, it's breaking a chemical bond that releases energy, separates a phosphate radical that converts ATP to adenosine diphosphate (ADP).

ADP is quickly reverted to ATP by receiving energy from food oxidation.

ATP is made up of three systems in muscles: the phosphate energy system, Glycogen-Lactic acid system, and the oxygen energy system. In that with the Lactic Acid Glycogen System, muscle cells separate glycogen into glucose, no needs oxygen, create ATP and lactic acid. In contrast, the oxygen system needs oxygen to oxidize sugar, protein and fat nutrients to generate energy. Sugar oxidation as sugar hydrolysis in the lactic acid system but with oxygen, causes lactic acid to continue oxidizing to $CO_2$ and water.

Therefore, when the body does strenuous exercise, people get sick, the elderly are weak, blood circulation is poor, and oxygen will not be sufficiently supplied to the nutrient oxidation and will produce lactic acid.

Lactic acid is a substance that causes fatigue, muscle aches and, worse, an acid environment in the body. When blood circulation is poor, $CO_2$ is a product of oxidation from cellular and is stagnant in all blood vessels, contributing to the formation of an acidic environment for the body by the formation of carbonic acid.

Protein, though not a major one, still contributes to energy supply. The metabolism proteins when the respiratory system provides oxygen deficiency also produces lactic acid which creates an acidic environment. When excessively eating protein, the protein will break down into urea and uric acid which create an acidic environment.

In fact, many studies have shown that our health depends very much on the pH of the body. For an immune system, self-repair, and to enzymes to work well, the body needs a mild alkalinity at a pH of 7.35. When the body is acidic, many diseases begin to appear: allergies, osteoporosis, obesity, diabetes, migraines, gout, stroke and cancer.

Otto Heinrich Warburg, a German biologist, Nobel laureate who won the Nobel Prize in 1931, invented a theory that cancer stemming from cell oxygen deficiency causes acidosis. In contrast, the body with high acidity causes hypoxia. All forms of cancer are characterized by two basic conditions: acidosis and hypoxia. Lack of oxygen and acidity are two sides of a coin; cancerous tissue is acidic, while healthy tissues are alkaline. The nature of cancer is due to genetic mutations, perhaps the acidic environment that supports this mutation.

The qigong practitioner often takes deep breaths, compressing the air; the air's solubility increases with the pressure, which in essence is an increase in oxygen exchange for the body, which is good for health. The metabolism of nutrients is like burning wood dry when it burns to create energy, whereas wet wood will produce smoke and product of burning is not finished, with the body they are lactic acid and free radicals.

2- Free radicals:

To this day, research by scientists has shown that the main culprit of aging and disease is free radicals. In the chemical structure, the atoms tend to bond firmly to each other so that the outer ring of electrons has 8 electrons, unlinked electrons always tend to be paired.

Due to chemical or radiation effects a broken chemical bond, each molecule holds an electron that creates a radical. Since solitary electrons are not in the form of pairs, they have very strong oxidation properties.

They always seek to grab the electrons that are missing from other molecules, and in turn, produce a chain of free radicals. In the body, they attack the cell membrane, protein molecules, and the cell nucleus etc., causing aging and cancer.

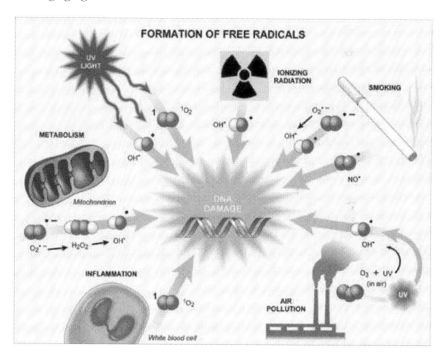

It is estimated that each cell suffers attack about 10,000 free radicals each day. So in the life of a person who lives to 70 years of age, about 17 tons of free radicals are created. (According to Wiki.).

### 3. Red meat and ion Fe in red meat:

University of California scientists has discovered that the human body detects red meat (pork, beef, and lamb...) as a strange substance and activates a toxic immune response. They discovered red meat containing a sugar called Neu5Gc, which when it was eaten by the body, triggers an immune response, producing antibodies that cause inflammation and ultimately lead to cancer.

Finally, when red meat is under high temperatures, such as grilled, fried, produces heterocyclic amino acids that also cause cancer.

Ion Fe is one of the very important minerals in the human body, especially in hemoglobin that transports oxygen in the blood to the tissues of the body. But too much iron in the diet can cause cirrhosis and liver cancer. Red meat is an iron-rich food. Iron compounds make the meat red. Iron is present in the cell as a transferrin that transports proteins in plasma to the receptors on the cell surface. When transferrin is saturated with iron, it activates cell proliferation. Another iron complex is hemosiderin that is released, which may create a series of adverse effects on liver cells. Excess diet Fe also stimulates oxidation to create free radicals.

Many vegetables and fruits have antioxidant active ingredients. Vitamin C is found in many common vegetables and fruits. Some vegetables, fruits, and especially oil-rich seeds contain vitamin E. More specifically, carotene-rich carrots, lycopene-rich tomatoes, onions, and garlic contain lots of allicin, ginger contains a lot of zingerol, tea contains dissolved tannins containing catechins (EGCG), and turmeric with curcumin etc.

Many research papers also suggest that cancer cells thrive in acidic environments. A meat-based diet create acidic, so it is better to eat fish and chicken than eating beef or pork. Meat also contains antibiotics for cattle, growth hormones and parasites. All are harmful, especially to cancer patients. Instead, a diet of 80% of fresh vegetables and fruit juices, whole grains, seeds and some fruits will put the body into an alkaline environment. About 20% can be cooked food, including beans. Fresh vegetable juice provides live enzymes that are easily absorbed and transferred to cells within 15 minutes to nourish and promote growth healthy cells. To have live enzymes, drink fresh vegetable juice (most vegetables including bean sprouts) and eat raw vegetables 2 or 3 times a day. Do not cook fresh vegetables because it loses many vitamins and enzymes which are destroyed at a temperature of 104 degrees F (40 degrees C). Protein in meat is difficult to digest and requires a lot of digestive enzymes. Undigested meat lying in the intestine will rot and lead to more toxic accumulation. Cancer cells have a hard protein shell. If you refrain or eat less meat, your body will release more enzymes to attack the protein coating of cancer cells and help the macrophage kill the cancer cells. Avoid coffee and chocolate because it contains high levels of caffeine. Drinking green tea is a better alternative, it also has anti-cancer properties. It is best to use purified water to avoid the toxins and heavy metals present in tap water. Distilled water is acidic, so do not drink it. Cancer is a disease of mind, body, and spirit. A dynamic life and active spirit will help cancer patients win the war against this disease and live longer.

As such, eat lots of vegetables, use plant protein as substitutes for animal protein, especially red meat, which eliminates the cause of acidic environment, removes excess of Fe ions in the diet, and eliminate the causes of free radicals and irritation. That is conditions and the risk factor causing cancer. In addition, combined with a diet rich in fresh vegetables, fruits and tubers containing vitamins C, vitamin E, β-carotene, polyphenols, flavonoids, selenium minerals, etc. All are functional foods. They are not only for the body but also the antioxidants, anti-free radical, anti-aging, and disease.

******

I write this article for my friend and for all others people including me. I have wide knowledge in many areas. However, just like many other people, there are several things that I know are not good but I still indulge in. These are not just eating habits but eating is also a passion and enjoyment. Good eating habit is an important part of a happy life.

At the moment I have noticed and controlled my eating habit but I'm not a complete vegetarian yet. I understand that if I don't follow this advice, I am a fool. So I find myself trying a strict diet plan because the failure of this means deteriorating health which would mean all is lost!

3-13-2017

# Vegetarian, what to eat and how to eat to fight cancer?

In the book, Vegetarianism to Prevent Cancer, which I gave my friend, had a story about Dr. Anthony Sattinaro, director of a large hospital in Philadelphia (USA). He had testicular cancer, prostate cancer (grade IV) and rib cancer. In three weeks he had to go to the operating table three times, cut off testicle, prostate, and finish with an examination of bone. According to modern medicine, he was only able to live a short time. But then, by chance, he was fasting and as a result, he recovered from illness.

He rewrote his story and it was published in Paris Match Magazine 10-1982 (France); Life Magazine 8-1982 (USA); Journal of Atarashiki Sekaia 10-1982 (Japan), and Newspaper "Đại đoàn kết" 11-1988 (Vietnam).

Anthony Sattinaro's father in Long Beach had just died of cancer. After attending funerals; on his way back to Philadelphia, he met two young men with long hair covering ears. They begged for a ride with him. The story had Eastern spirituality color, he hated such young men but does not know why he would let them ride with him this time, and he thought that two men had a "mission" to rescue him.

When talking, the two young men told him that they had graduated from a cooking class. He couldn't hide his sadness, he had just buried his father died who died of cancer. In turn, he knew he will also dying of cancer.

He was surprised when one of the two young men said he did not need to die, cancer was not difficult to cure, just change the way of eating, and remove animal food. A doctor, director of a hospital in the United States, with the most developed Western medicine, first heard this from the mouth of a boy he could not believe it. And then, when he got home, he received a book about the magic ability of the cure for cancer by the method "macrobiotic" from two young men. And then, in a no way out, overcoming his suspicion, and of his colleague in the hospital, he found the place of Denny Waxman, an OHSAWA method advocate in Philadelphia. But he still cannot help thinking that he had entrusted his life to a group of ignorant Eastern physicians!

Because he had Type IV cancer, in his meal, the Waxman family completely eliminate some of his favorite foods such as meat, milk, and processed starches, etc. He only ate 50-60% of cups, 25% of vegetables, 15% of beans and seaweed, the rest is miso and spices.

After a few weeks, he wrote: "the play of theater begins". One morning, he reached over to take the painkillers, and he was surprised to realize he had no pain at all. "It's like having someone help me take off my shirt that is too tight". And then after 13 months of vegetarian diet, he was completely cured!

******

In the view of Western medicine, the menu of Dr. Anthony Sattinaro as described above would not only fail to cure cancer but it would also mean that Dr. Anthony would die as a result of the lack of proteins in his meals.

Cellular ribosomes requires different amino acids for protein biosynthesis. Deficiency of any amino acid means protein cannot be formed. Of these, about 8 amino acids that the human body does not synthesize are called essential amino acids. They are supplied by the food we eat. If your diet lacks one of these 8 important nutrients, it can lead to some serious diseases. In the mind of most people as well as of Western medicine, vegetable proteins often lack essential amino acids.

But in fact, the vegetarians are not only healthy but are also cured of many diseases, including cancer. This is simply because eating a type food from a plant may lack some essential amino acids, but if you eat a variety, they will not lack.

The World Health Organization (WHO) recommends that adults take 5% of daily calories from protein. This amount of protein is easily achieved by eating raw starch (brown rice) and vegetables. Children at the highest development stage need mother's milk containing 5% protein. Compared to rice which contains 8% protein, corn has 11%, oatmeal has 15%, and bean has 27%. As such, protein deficiency is unlikely to occur if adults eat vegetables and unprocessed cereals. So, the vegetarian advocates claim that the American Heart Association (AHA) statement is often quoted, "but incorrect". They wrote that in the plant proteins "most of them lack one.

29

Or many essential amino acids and are, therefore, considered incomplete proteins. "

In 1952, William Rose and his colleagues identified human requirements for eight essential amino acids, giving the "minimum amino acid requirements" of a body and then doubling as considered an "absolutely safe dose". By calculating a number of essential amino acids supplied by the raw starch and comparing these values with the substances identified by Rose, the results show that any combination of the plant foods provided Amino acids all exceed the recommended requirement.

Therefore, the main cause of the diseases of modern times is mainly as a result of the development. Life is rich and leisurely. People eat a lot more but work less. Nutrition that exceeds body needs does not completely metabolize and only accumulate as fat, an excess of protein, and create many toxic substances. All of them are the causes of all kinds of diseases.

******

However, based on this fact, researchers also recommended that vegetarians can avoid anemia resulting from iron deficiency by eating more fruits and vegetables that are high in vitamin C. Vitamin C increases absorption of iron and resist the inhibition iron absorption of phytic acid, oxalic acid, tannic acid ...

Pregnant women, nursing mothers, infants, teenagers, athletes or people with high blood loss should use iron supplements. Vitamin B12 deficiency can also occur in absolute vegetarians because of plant foods that lack vitamin B12. This vitamin is recommended for pregnant women who are vegetarians. The same applies to breast-feeding women and especially the elderly (because they often reduce their absorption of vitamin B12.) Zinc deficiency can also occur in vegetarians. Zinc in plant foods is less absorbed by phytic acid, oxalates, fiber, and soy protein, and there is a risk of zinc deficiency among older adults (whether vegetarian or not). Take tablets containing zinc.

When cooking, it is important to note that plant seeds have the mechanism of self-protection inhibits germination to germinate in appropriate seasons, with two chemicals is abscisic acid and phytic acid present in the bran.

These two substances are harmful to health. So scientists advise us to "turn on the switch" for germinated brown rice by submerging it, but only to the "Germination mode." At this time, the poisonous ingredient inside the seed has been changed to be safe for human consumption. Then the enzymes that sleep in the rice grains at this state are stimulated to function and provide maximum nutrients.

Nutritionists also advise on the need to eat complete foods. These are foods that Nature bestowed upon mankind, such as bran, cereals, bulbs, and roots of vegetables; the need to eat raw foods whenever possible to conserve vitamins and active ingredients. Tomatoes and carrots need to be cooked with some oil to dissolve lycopene and carotene.

******

Vegetables, bulbs, and fruits have the effect of preventing and fighting cancer because they contain vitamins and active substances with resistance to mutations, antioxidants, inhibit disease onset and isolate cancer cells against the spread of the disease.

Vitamin C dissolved in water should strongly destroy the radicals dissolved in the water phase; Vitamin E dissolved in oil will collect and destroy free radicals in the lipids. Carotenoids are a "drink" of free oxygen, 20 times more potent than vitamin E.

A solution of crushed eggplant and crushed amaranth was found to be strongest against the mutation. A solution of crushed amaranth killed cancer cells, particularly breast cancer, liver cancer, and lung cancer. Beetroot is considered one of the vegetables that is most effective in treating leukemia and cancer. Betaine, an amino acid that has strong anti-cancer properties, is also a potent anti-inflammatory and anti-oxidant.

Rudolf Breuss, an Austrian researcher, used fruit juice: Beetroot (55%), carrots (20%), celery (20%), potatoes (3%), white cabbage (2%) and gave his patients drink every day, he helped more than 45,000 people with cancer and other incurable diseases to treat the disease effectively. The patients that drunk that juice mixture for 42 consecutive days showed the evidence of their cancer cells thoroughly destroyed. (http://www.baomoi.com/ )

20-3-2017

# Once Again, Let's Talk About Vegetarian Diet to Fight Cancer

## (When the author was reading the information about Actor DUY THANH who was suffering from cancer and waiting to die)

People's thinking habits follow inertia, in the usual sense, follow the crowd. That is why it is hard for people to believe in the differences, contrary to common sense, especially "anti-science". But if science is understood, there will be extraordinary phenomena but they are true. Only knowledgeable scientists will recognize, study, explain, and when they prove successful, it means, they have promoted the science of development, given humanity new knowledge. For example, the invention of antimatter, the speed of light is constant, intermittent emission energy, mass is bending space-time, etc.

Talk outside the main content a little I want to talk that vegetarian diets against cancer also have similarities. Modern medicine is yet to concede that vegetarian diet can cure cancer. While in fact, many witnesses have proved that Vegetarian diet can cure cancer. Why is it that the World's Medicine is yet to study and apply it?

So it is heartbreaking to read the newspaper's coverage that Actor Duy Thanh, after a period of time has been positively treated by modern Medicine at the hospital, yet he was still at the stage where he was just waiting to die.

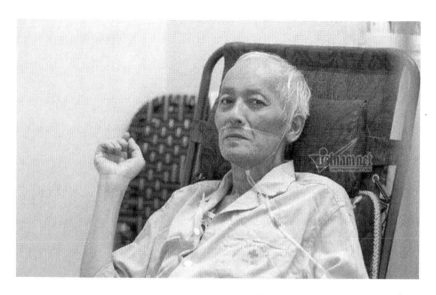

*(Actor Duy Thanh)*

So I want to tell a story shared by many on their personal web pages about a former staff member at 108 Army Medical Institute who had cancer. He studied the "macrobiotic" method and cured himself before curing many other people. He wanted to popularize his healing methods so that everyone could apply them.

That is Mr. Nguyen Minh Tuan (72 years old), a former staff of Military Hospital 108, and the son of the director of Military Hospital 108 in the 60s.

From self-healing, Mr. Tuan studied macrobiotic method of Oshawa. He said that since 1983, doctors had known that he had cancer at a late stage. Two large tumors in the lungs. Working in the Hospital 108, he had access to all conditions for treatment. But in the course of treatment, the chief of the Oriental Medicine Department of the Hospital 108 showed him how to treat cancer by "hunger-strike" and Macrobiotic method. At that time, he had only very few evidence but he said, doesn't understand why he had a strong belief in that method and he decided to follow it.

Back then, there were many people stopping him. Even until now, still many nutritional experts believe that cancer cure by fasting, eating brown rice and sesame salt is a scam and unscientific, that time, more than 30 years ago, could anyone agree with him?

But he was resolute please leave the hospital, go home for self-healing.

But he resolutely asked to leave the hospital to go home for self-healing. He left the hospital on August 20, 1983. The papers indicate that he had cancerous tumors in lobes of the right lung. The hospital convinced him to continue with the treatment, but he refused to continue with medication, or even performing tests for monitoring and treatment. He eagerly applied to leave the hospital to treat himself and took responsibility for his illness.

After trying their best to convince him, the doctors finally accepted to release him. He had decided to go away no one in Vietnam had ever gone although the method was becoming popular in the rest of the world at that time.

His father was the director 108 military hospitals, later Director of Viet Tiep Hai Phong Hospital. When he found out he was sick, of course, his father advised him to follow the Western Medicine. But when he presented his ideas, his father respected his choice even though he did not believe in it. He ate 100%: brown rice and sesame salt, ate only two meals a day, morning and afternoon, no dinner. On Sundays, he did not eat at all.

After 4 months, he had lost 25 kgs in weights. Seeing his health deteriorate, His hospital colleagues must come to his home, forcing him to go to the hospital. He was forced to obey orders. But in the hospital, he decided not to take a pill, refuse biopsy test. He only allowed doctors to film his lungs.

Results X-ray shows that the tumor, like a chicken egg in his lungs, has disappeared completely. The doctors were surprised. His father came to the hospital to see X-ray film and was equally shocked. Though very happy that his son was far away from death, his father remained silent. Everyone was happy, only he understood that this was only like as cutting the top of the tree, the root of the disease is really scary.

He explained that he had resolutely chosen fasting and "macrobiotic" methods. According to him, understanding this method is very simple. For example, a tree that is not watered, not fertilized, will not be green. The animal is also similar, without food it will be stunted and cannot grow. This is the same case for humans.

No one can live without food or drinks. From that simple principle, we can understand that if the disease is not nourished it will also die. The germ is the same. All plants, animals, and diseases will die when they are not provided with nutrition.

If we proceed to cleanse the blood and provide a good amount of vegetable protein to the body, it will keep the blood and the body in good condition. Eating brown rice and sesame salt is good for that. After fasting and "hunger strike" in a suitable time, the blood changes. At this time, the human body is a clean environment, so bacteria and tumors have no nutrients to live on.

And he had been eating brown rice and sesame salt for more than 30 years he kept a frugal lifestyle. The result is that up to date he is still healthy, what a clever mind!

He thinks everyone can apply this method, but like western medicine, must be started early to bring efficiency. If the patient's illness is too severe, it cannot work.

Before "hunger-strike", it is necessary to wash the intestines taking diluted porridge. The first day he took three bowls of porridge in place of each meal. 2nd day halved the amount of porridge compared to the first day, the third day, took even less diluted porridge.

The patient must ensure that nothing is left in the colon before starting "hunger-strike". During these three days, eat another 50 grams of sesame per day to increase laxative. During the process of "hunger-strike," don't eat any kind of food, except filtered water. When doing "hunger-strike" to the maximum threshold, the patient may not bear it, and may start to eat again. The patient starts to drink from the water of brown rice roasted, and finally eating rice.

The problem with "hunger-strike" as a tool against cancer is that patients can die of hunger before dying of cancer? He said that people die of hunger only when there is no nutrient in the body. The "hunger-strike" in this case is under control, of course, it depends on how fat or skinny one is to determine takes for fasting to be appropriate.

The special thing that he remind patients undergoing "hunger strike" is that when eating back, they have to chew all the food carefully. Chewing like that not just help the sick to swallow easily, it is also an activity that helps stimulates salivation, for nutrition to be absorbed into the stomach wall in the most effective way, providing enough nutrition for the body. Now, after 30 years of implementation "Macrobiotic" method to cure cancer, he still eats meat and fish occasionally but eats only a small portion, only about 10% of the food intake. He can eat 1-2 times a week.

He regrets that until now, this method has not been studied in detail in Vietnam although it has helped a lot of people get cured. In 2007, Vietnam Union of Science and Technology Associations held a workshop on nutrition. He was invited to present at this workshop. Of course, there were many people in the conference who said that, his story was a scam, but there are also people who said that it needed to be studied in detail and based on specific information and evidence about people who have been cured of cancer, through the medical records that he together with a doctor at the Children's Institute brought to present.

The scientists objected is due to the one-sided view. Because of this method, there are very scientific explanations that he has presented. And there are also scientists had analyzed the nutrition content of brown rice. Specific, bran of brown rice contains 120 antioxidants such as CoQ10, alpha-lipoic acid, oligomeric proanthocyanidins, SOD, tocopherol and tocotrienol, IP6 (inositol hexaphosphate), glutathione, carotenoids, selenium, phytosterols, lutein, and lycopene.

Therefore, brown rice has excellent effects in protecting the body against free radicals, supporting cancer treatment. IP6 contained in brown rice is a substance that has powerful anti-cancer activity, especially against cancer cells in the liver and intestines. Sesame salt, (use coarse salt) unrefined to keep the minerals needed for the body, sesame contains large amounts of calcium, iron, and other nutrients and is an excellent source of vegetable oil that cannot produce cholesterol.

He asserted that this is not a deceptive or unscientific method as people think. But to successfully treat cancer, patients should have the determination and very much perseverance.

Los Angeles

*26-8-2017*

# The deepest essence of anti-cancer by vegetarianism method

## (Apply a diet of which the essential amino acids, not excess compared to body needs)

According to Vietnam Net, a National Assembly official said at a meeting in Vietnam: "Each year, cancer is responsible for about 70,000 deaths and more than 200,000 new cases reported are caused by unsafe food."

But health minister Nguyen Thi Kim Tien said, "There are no grounds to say that many cancer patients die because of food safety."

The answer surprised many, many people wrote articles to ridicule the knowledge of the minister. But Ms. Tien is Associate Professor Ph.D. of medicine, a former director of Pasteur Institute Ho Chi Minh City, head of the subject at the University of Medicine and Pharmacy HCM city.

Ms. Tien explained:

"The ministry invited experts from within and even outside the country to find out the causes of cancer deaths. The results show that leading causes of cancer are acute and chronic infections. For example, hepatitis B and hepatitis C which causes chronic hepatitis, liver cancer."

If well understood, what the minister said right.

The case of food poisoning is acute, the patient has to be taken to the emergency room for quick treatment. Failure of this may mean death.

Cancer is a genetic mutation resulting from several factors such as radiation, free radicals (by metabolism), toxins (smoking, food containing pesticides, and mold), etc.

These are factors that may not be toxic enough to kill the body cells but causes mutation instead.

The cell changes and starts growing out of control. It does not follow Apoptosis (a process of programmed growth that occurs in multicellular organisms,) causing cancerous tumors.

These chemicals that cause mutations may have chemical properties that interact with DNA functional groups, distort the normal programming of GOT, "The creator of the universe". There is documentation that people with hepatitis B and eat moldy food containing aflatoxin will increase the risk of cancer 60 times higher than people with - hepatitis B only.

******

About the cause of cancer, people's perceptions are generally clear and consistent. On treatment, with cancer at the stage of development, the Medicine still is impotent. But there are cancer patients when trying to use the informal treatments that have cured the disease but have not been recognized by modern medicine. These are methods that have not been studied and proven clinically too applicable for the treatment of cancer.

The method has got more than enough mentions. There are many witnesses for this "macrobiotic" method. It involves the use of vegetarian food, and more positive, it includes "hunger strike" in the suitable time. The basis of the method is the reasoning that cutting the nutrient source from the tumor destroys it completely.

According to another article on Vietnam Net, Associate Prof. Dr. Nguyen Thi Lam, Deputy Director of National Institute of Nutrition said:

"Many cancer patients think that they do not eat to heal because they are afraid that cancer cells will develop if they eat a lot. This is a very wrong concept. Many patients suffering from the long-term diet have ended up dead as a result of deteriorating health before dying of cancer."

Associate Prof. Dr. Lam recommends that patients with cancer need to eat enough foods with adequate vitamins and minerals so that the body is able to fight off the destruction of cancer cells. Need to eat the full range of powders, sugar, protein, and fat etc. in vegetables, meat, and fish".

Dr. Pham Cam Phuong, deputy director of the Center for Nuclear Medicine and Oncology, Bach Mai Hospital, also said that if for cancer only, and the patient is not suffering from combined diseases such as diabetes, hyperlipidemia ... Do not diet:

"Do not think that if you do not eat, then the tumor does not grow, this is completely wrong. The tumor still develops and take the substances of your body whether you eat or not. If the patient does not eat or drink, it will be depleted, exhausted due to cancer, not healthy enough to go for the follow-up therapies to reduce the risk of cancer and prevent metastasis."

If you take the words of the two persons above, patients with cancer will get cured, there is nothing to add on this. But in reality, with the active treatment of modern medicine, they still die, like actor Duy Thanh a few days ago also shared online, now dead. On the contrary, with the method which the modern medical still considered "anti-common arguments", "anti-Medical", in fact, it has saved many cancer patients when the hospital was helpless, helping them to regain life!

Two medical specialists above were wrong, speaking following common theories, like parrots. Actually, the conventional method of treatment is helpless if the cancer has developed. People need to look wider into fact, need to recognize and research better and appreciate the unconventional treatment methods. Two people above also need to understand the distinction, the cancer patients using vegetarian method (eat vegetable protein instead of animal protein) combined with a "hunger strike" in a suitable time, not what they describe as a hunger strike to death!

I myself can also be a witness. On my face, I had a mole just under the left eye four years ago. Suddenly, I saw it become itchy and start growing. I decided to go for a test to see if the mole was turning into melanoma? But then I remember the story I used to buy a book about vegetarian method and combined with a "hunger strike" in a suitable time to cure cancer. This is the book I used to share with the sick and advise them to apply. After reading that book, I knew tumor cells grow faster than normal cells and need more nutrient to support this rapid growth. What it needs most is the "material" to grow like people need materials to build a house. That material is animal protein. Think so, I decided to try "hunger strike", and imitate Ms. Vu Thi Hoa, who could see and communicate with the soul of the dead. As such, I only drunk coconut water. My health did not deteriorate, it was normal, although I feel the body is empty and light in weight. But know melanoma is a dangerous type of cancer. I didn't know if I was really sick or not. But think of it this way, it is better to prevent it with a hunger strike. And then the miracle happened. After about 10 days, I talk with my nephew: "Have a look, how is my mole changing?" "I see the edge of it is detaching out". I am happy to have results but I was also frightened, "was it really cancer?" I was more determined. Finally, after a few more days, I continued to drink coconut water and the mole was gone. How aghast! I believe it is a melanoma because at the bottom of my neck there was a big mole that was an ordinary mole, it is still intact, unaffected by eating!

So wonderful, the method of "hunger strike" just as I thought, just as the document was written, it is capable of destroying cancer tumor!

******

One rare thing happened, it was not intentional but is evidence to researchers recognize how is Human survival dependent into nutrition?

There is a story posted in the popular newspapers in Vietnam. In 1981, 10 Irish prisoners from the Republican Army (IRA) went on a hunger strike. 9 out of 10 men starved after between 57 and 73 days (average 61.6 days) and lost about 40% of their body weight. Doctors found that when people are hungry, the body's stored protein is generally protected. So as to have the energy to live, the body mainly uses energy from fat reserves. It is estimated that by the time of the death, hunger strikers lose 94% of their fat, but only 19% of the protein is lost. They died because they ran out of fat, not because they ran out of protein. This is the scientific basis for the removal of animal protein from the diet, to kill the cancerous tumor by way for hungry tumor for it to die. This approach cannot be too dangerous for the body to cope. If the body can be weak due to lack of protein but cancerous cells are killed. As the result, we are faced with an option between being weak and facing death. Which one will you choose? Of course people only use the method of "hunger strike" in a suitable time to overcome the status of dangerous tumors develop. In fact, with the vegetarian diet, the body still get all the nutrients. Yes, it is difficult to change your diet and habits all at once, but it is something any of us can do. I did it, so can you?

******

According to the document on cancer at Johns Hopkins Hospital, Baltimore, USA, answering the question, "What are living by cancer cells?"

They write: "Sugar is a carcinogen - cutting off sugar is cutting an important food supply for cancer cells". In my opinion, sugar is only an energy-producing substance for the tumor, it acts like gasoline for a car. Cutting off sugar is important, but I think, you should target to cut the source of the building material to the tumor. This is more important. That is protein.

Tumors need to have proteins to form cells. These are provided from functional proteins formed by protein synthesis in cells from amino acids coming from the nutrient source.

Activated amino acids bind to transport RNA (tRNA), which are then linked together to the protein through the process Code translation (ribosome binding to the mRNA molecule) in accordance with the template that is transcribed to form the mRNA from DNA. So the material builds up in the cell are Amino Acids. When both sources of animal protein and vegetable protein are available. But why is it that eating vegetable protein is effective against cancer? In my opinion, simply because vegetable protein have essential amino acids but low in quantity, not even enough for the body, what about the tumor that needs it in vast amounts?

So, is the essential amino acids are missing, where will the tumor get the protein to form and grow? We need have to understand missing an essential amino acid is all whole chain of proteins that cannot be formed during protein synthesis in the cell. Protein is not formed, there will be no material for the tumor to develop.

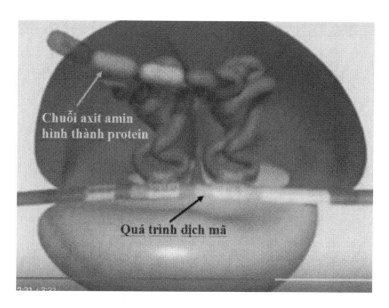

Chuỗi axit amin
hình thành protein

Quá trình dịch mã

(The Process translation for protein synthesis)

This is what makes the tumor die by its greediness! Interestingly, it is because the essential amino acid of vegetable protein is low, so is a weapon for killing cancer. It is like poverty that has good points because it forces people to eat a healthy diet, to avoid illness due to overeating.

Now there is a lot of information on the net, you have many choices but choosing right is not easy. You need to understand comprehensively and deeply.

My friend suffering from liver cancer changed to become a vegetarian completely. He followed my instructions carefully. Three months after surgery, he went back to the clinic at the hospital for examination. The doctor could no longer see any cancer tumors. At the same time but not following the vegetarian diet as he did before, he went to the clinic after being infected with the hepatitis B virus. From the absence of any tumor, the doctor said he had four tumors liver!

And even more happy when I saw, on facebook, my friend that just announced this:

"For the first nine months of treatment, the AFP index was 6.8 below the normal range of 10. I'm so happy to reward myself with 2 cans of 333 ".

So diets have prevented the growth of cancer cells.

*4-11-2017*

# PART II: MACROBIOTIC DIET AND GENERAL SCIENCE

*(So, from the stories told, we see: the Macrobiotic diet of George Ohsawa, the sources of nutrients, metabolism in the body, nutritional needs of the body and of cancer tumors, free radicals, etc. are related to the cause of cancer and the cure for cancer. So following this, we dig deeper on the scientific basis of these claims).*

# George Ohsawa and His macrobiotic diet

*(From Wikipedia, the free encyclopedia)*

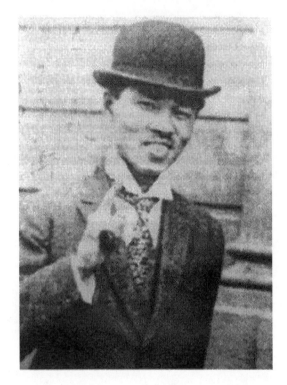

*(George Ohsawa, October 18, 1893 – April 23, 1966)*

George Ohsawa, born in Nyoichi Sakurazawa, (October 18, 1893 – April 23, 1966), was the founder of the Macrobiotic diet and philosophy. He was born in a poor samurai family in Shingu City Wakayama pref Japan.

George Ohsawa introduced the oriental concept of health to Westerners in the mid-20th century.

The gradual introduction of sugar into the Japanese diet brought in its wake the beginning of Western diseases, which were abandoned as incurable by the Western doctors. Dr. Sagen Ishizuka, a Japanese practitioner became famous because thousands of patients had been cured by him (through traditional use of food) after they were abandoned as incurable by the new medicine of the West.

Ohsawa states in his books that he cured himself of tuberculosis at age 19 by applying the ancient concept of yin and yang that originated in China, as well as the teachings of Sagen Ishizuka.

He traveled to Europe; particularly Paris in France where he began to spread his philosophy. After several years, he returned to Japan to start a foundation, and gather recruits for his now formalized philosophy. In 1931, he published The Unique Principle explaining the yin and yang order of the universe.

Macrobiotic diet

*"A macrobiotic diet (or macrobiotics) is a fad diet fixed on ideas about types of food drawn from Zen Buddhism. The diet attempts to balance the supposed yin and yang elements of food and cookware. Major principles of macrobiotic diets are to reduce animal product, eat locally grown foods that are in season, and consume meals in moderation.*

*A macrobiotic diet is helpful for people with cancer and other chronic diseases, although there is no good evidence to support such recommendations. Neither the American Cancer Society nor Cancer Research UK recommends adopted the diet. Suggestions that a macrobiotic diet improves cardiovascular disease and diabetes as explained by the diet being, in part, consistent with science-based dietary approaches to disease prevention.*

*Macrobiotic diets are based on the concept of balancing yin and yang."*

**Source:** https://en.wikipedia.org/wiki/Macrobiotic_diet

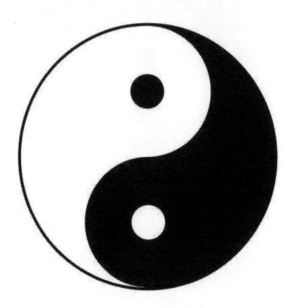

(Macrobiotic diets are based on the concept of balancing yin and yang)

Macrobiotics emphasizes locally grown whole grain cereals, pulses (legumes), vegetables, seaweed, fermented soy products and fruit, combined into meals according to the ancient Chinese principle of balance known as yin and yang. Whole grains and whole-grain products such as brown rice and buckwheat pasta (soba), a variety of cooked and raw vegetables, beans and bean products, mild natural seasonings, fish, nuts, and seeds, mild (non-stimulating) beverages such as bancha twig tea and fruit are recommended.

Some Macrobiotic proponents, including George Ohsawa, stress the fact that yin and yang are relative qualities that can only be determined in a comparison. All food is considered to have both properties, with one dominating. Foods with yang qualities are considered compact, dense, heavy, hot, whereas those with yin qualities are considered expansive, light, cold, and diffuse. However, these terms are relative; "yangness" or "yinness" is only discussed in relation to other foods.

Brown rice and other whole grains such as barley, millet, oats, quinoa, spelt, rye, and teff are considered by macrobiotics to be the foods in which yin and yang are closest to being in balance. Therefore, lists of macrobiotic foods that determine a food as yin or yang generally compare them to whole grains.

# Metabolism in the body

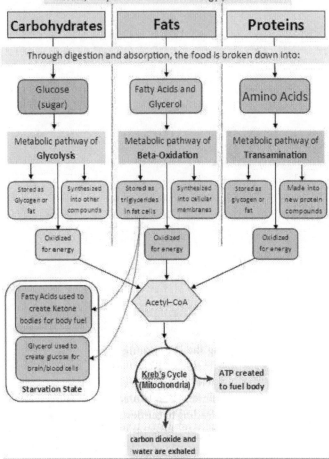

In the **fed** state, nutrients are stored; In the **fasting** state, they are oxidized for energy production

| Carbohydrates | Fats | Proteins |

Through digestion and absorption, the food is broken down into:

| Glucose (sugar) | Fatty Acids and Glycerol | Amino Acids |

| Metabolic pathway of Glycolysis | Metabolic pathway of Beta-Oxidation | Metabolic pathway of Transamination |

| Stored as Glycogen or fat | Synthesized into other compounds | Stored as triglycerides in fat cells | Synthesized into cellular membranes | Stored as glycogen or fat | Made into new protein compounds |

| Oxidized for energy | Oxidized for energy | Oxidized for energy |

Fatty Acids used to create Ketone bodies for body fuel

Glycerol used to create glucose for brain/blood cells

**Starvation State**

Acetyl-CoA

Kreb's Cycle (Mitochondria) → ATP created to fuel body

carbon dioxide and water are exhaled

Most of the time, metabolism works well. But sometimes a person's metabolism can cause major mayhem in the form of a metabolic disorder. In a broad sense, a metabolic disorder is any disease that is caused by an abnormal chemical reaction in the body's cells.

Most disorders of metabolism involve either abnormal levels of enzymes or hormones or problems with how those enzymes or hormones work. When the metabolism of body chemicals is blocked or defective, it can cause a buildup of toxic substances in the body or a lack of substances needed for normal body function, either of which can cause serious symptoms.

Metabolic diseases and conditions include:

Hyperthyroidism. Hyperthyroidism is caused by an overactive thyroid gland. It causes symptoms such as weight loss, increased heart rate and blood pressure, protruding eyes, and a swelling in the neck from an enlarged thyroid (goiter). The disease may be controlled with medicines or through surgery or radiation treatments.

Hypothyroidism is caused by a nonexistent or underactive thyroid gland. Untreated hypothyroidism can lead to brain and growth problems in infants and children. Hypothyroidism slows body processes and causes tiredness, slow heart rate, weight gain, and constipation. Teens who have it can be treated with oral thyroid hormone.

Metabolic diseases that are inherited are called inborn errors of metabolism. When babies are born, they're tested for many of these. Inborn errors of metabolism include galactosemia (babies born with this do not have enough of the enzyme that breaks down the sugar in milk, called galactose) and phenylketonuria (this is due to a defect in the enzyme that breaks down the amino acid phenylalanine, needed for normal growth and protein production). Inborn errors of metabolism can sometimes lead to serious problems if they're not controlled with diet or medicine from an early age.

Type 1 diabetes. Type 1 diabetes happens when the pancreas doesn't make and secrete enough insulin. Symptoms of this disease include excessive thirst and peeing, hunger, and weight loss. Over time, the disease can cause kidney problems, pain due to nerve damage, blindness, and heart and blood vessel disease. Teens with type 1 diabetes need regular insulin injections and should control their blood sugar levels to reduce the risk of developing problems from diabetes.

Type 2 diabetes. Type 2 diabetes happens when the body can't respond normally to insulin. Symptoms are similar to those of type 1 diabetes. Many children and teens who develop type 2 diabetes are overweight, and this is thought to play a role in their decreased responsiveness to insulin. Some teens can be treated successfully with dietary changes, exercise, and oral medicine; others will need insulin injections. Controlling blood sugar levels reduces the risk of developing the same kinds of long-term health problems that happen with type 1 diabetes.

Digestion of food

Digestion is a necessary first step for all foods. Digestion results in the formation of smaller molecules that are able to pass through that lining and enter the person's bloodstream. It includes simple sugars (formed by the breakdown of complex carbohydrates), glycerol and fatty acids (formed by the breakdown of lipids), and amino acids (formed by the breakdown of proteins). Cells use substances in the metabolic pool as building materials.

Cellular metabolism

Substances that make up the metabolic pool are transported to individual cells by the bloodstream. They pass through cell membranes and enter the cell interior. Once inside a cell, a compound undergoes further metabolism, usually in a series of chemical reactions. For example, a sugar molecule is broken down inside a cell into carbon dioxide and water, with the release of energy. But that process does not occur in a single step. Instead, it takes about two dozen separate chemical reactions to convert the sugar molecule to its final products.

The purpose of these reactions is to release energy stored in the sugar molecule. To explain that process, one must know that a sugar molecule consists of carbon, hydrogen, and oxygen atoms held together by means of chemical bonds. A chemical bond is a force of attraction between two atoms. That force of attraction is a form of energy. A sugar molecule with two dozen chemical bonds can be thought of as containing two dozen tiny units of energy. Each time a chemical bond is broken, one unit of energy is set free.

Cells have evolved remarkable methods for capturing and storing the energy released in catabolic reactions. Those methods make use of very special chemical compounds, known as energy carriers. An example of such compounds is adenosine triphosphate generally known as ATP. ATP is formed when adenosine diphosphate (ADP) combines with a phosphate group. The following equation represents that change:

$$ADP + P \rightarrow ATP$$

ADP will combine with a phosphate group only if energy is added to it. In cells, that energy comes from the catabolism of compounds such as sugars, glycerol, and fatty acids.

Metabolism can be conveniently divided into two categories:

Catabolism - the breakdown of molecules to obtain energy.

Anabolism - the synthesis of all compounds needed by the cells.

The ATP molecule formed in this way, then, has taken up the energy previously stored in the sugar molecule. Whenever a cell needs energy for some process, it can obtain it from an ATP molecule.

The reverse of the process shown above also takes place inside cells. That is, energy from an ATP molecule can be used to put simpler molecules together to make more complex molecules. For example, suppose that a cell needs to repair a break in its cell wall. To do so, it will need to produce new protein molecules. Those protein molecules can be made from amino acids in the metabolic pool. A protein molecule consists of hundreds or thousands of amino acid molecules joined to each other.

The energy needed to form all the new chemical bonds needed to hold the amino acid units together comes from ATP molecules.

Metabolism is closely linked to nutrition.

Essential nutrients supply energy (calories) and supply the necessary chemicals, which the body itself cannot synthesize like oxygen, nitrogen, carbon, hydrogen, sulfur, phosphorus, and around 20 other inorganic elements. The major elements are supplied in carbohydrates, lipids, and protein. In addition, vitamins, minerals, and water are necessary.

*"Foods supply carbohydrates in three forms: starch, sugar, and cellulose (fiber). Body tissues depend on glucose for all activities. The overall reaction to the combustion of glucose is written as:*

$$C_6H_{12}O_6 + 6\ O_2 \rightarrow 6\ CO_2 + 6\ H_2O + energy$$

*Most people consume around half of their diet as carbohydrates. This comes from rice, wheat, bread, potatoes, pasta, macaroni etc.*

*\*\*\*\*\*\**

*Proteins are the main tissue builders in the body. They are part of every cell in the body. Proteins help in cell structure, functions, and hemoglobin formation to carry oxygen, enzymes to carry out vital reactions and a myriad of other functions in the body. Proteins are also vital in supplying nitrogen for DNA and RNA genetic material and energy production. Sugar addition in diet and its effect on appetite, fat breakdown, and energy metabolism.*

*Proteins are necessary for nutrition because they contain amino acids. Among the 20 or more amino acids, the human body is unable to synthesize 8 and these are called essential amino acids.*

*The essential amino acids include lysine, tryptophan, methionine, leucine, isoleucine, phenylalanine, valine, and threonine.*

*\*\*\*\*\*\**

*Fats are concentrated sources of energy. They produce twice as much energy as either carbohydrates or protein on a weight basis. The functions of fats include:*

*Helping to form the cellular structure; forming a protective cushion and insulation around vital organs; helping absorb fat-soluble vitamins, providing a reserve storage for energy. Essential fatty acids include unsaturated fatty acids like linoleic, linolenic, and arachidonic acids. These need to be taken in the diet. Saturated fats, along with cholesterol, have been implicated in arteriosclerosis and heart disease.*

*\*\*\*\*\*\**

*The minerals in foods do not contribute directly to energy needs but are important as body regulators and play a role in metabolic pathways of the body. More than 50 elements are found in the human body. About 25 elements have been found to be essential since a deficiency produces specific deficiency symptoms.*

*Important minerals include calcium, phosphorus, iron, sodium, potassium, chloride ions, copper, cobalt, manganese, zinc, magnesium, fluorine, and iodine."*

**Source:** https://www.news-medical.net/life-sciences/What-is-

Metabolism.aspx

\*\*\*\*\*\*

Vitamins are essential organic compounds that the human body cannot synthesize by itself and must, therefore, be present in the diet. Vitamins particularly important in metabolism include Vitamin A, B2 (riboflavin), Niacin or nicotinic acid, Pantothenic Acid etc. Metabolic pathways

The chemical reactions of metabolism are organized into metabolic pathways. These allow the basic chemicals from nutrition to be transformed through a series of steps into another chemical, by a sequence of enzymes.

Enzymes are crucial to metabolism because they allow organisms to drive desirable reactions that require energy. These reactions also are coupled with those that release.

# Free radicals

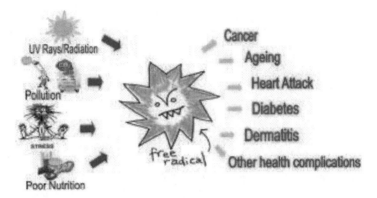

To this day, research by scientists has shown that the main culprit of aging and disease is free radicals.

In the chemical structure, the atoms tend to bond firmly to each other so that the outer ring of electrons has 8 electrons, and unlinked electrons always tend to be paired. Because of the chemical or radiation affect a broken chemical bond, each molecule holds an electron create a radical. Because solitary electrons are not in the form of pairs, so they have very strong oxidation properties. They always seek to grab the electrons that are missing from other molecules, and in turn, produce a chain of free radicals. They reactive even towards themselves: their molecules will often spontaneously dimerize or polymerize if they come in contact with each other. In chemical equations, free radicals are frequently denoted by a dot placed immediately to the right of the atomic symbol or molecular formula.

Example of a free radical is:

The hydroxyl radical (HO•), a molecule that has one unpaired electron on the oxygen atom. The two most important oxygen-centered free radicals are superoxide and hydroxyl radical. They derive from molecular oxygen under reducing conditions.

Chlorine gas can be broken down by ultraviolet light to form atomic chlorine radicals.

Free radicals may be created in a number of ways, including reactions at very low temperatures, or any process that puts enough energy into the parent molecule, such as ionizing radiation, heat, electrical discharges, electrolysis, and chemical reactions, also can affect breakup of larger molecules. Radicals are intermediate stages in many chemical reactions.

The formation of radicals may involve the breaking of covalent bonds by hemolysis, a process that requires significant amounts of energy. Such energies are known as homolytic bond dissociation energies.

The energy needed to break a specific bond (generally covalent) between two atoms known as bond energy. Likewise, radicals requiring more energy to form are less stable than those requiring less energy.

Radical formation through homolytic bond cleavage most often happens between two atoms of similar electronegativity; in organic chemistry, this is often between the O–O bonds in peroxide species or between O–N bonds. Radicals may also be formed by single-electron oxidation or reduction of an atom or molecule.

*"The unpaired electrons make free radicals highly chemically reactive towards other substances, or even towards themselves: their molecules will often spontaneously dimerize or polymerize if they come in contact with each other."*

Free radicals play an important role in many other chemical processes. In living organisms, the free radicals superoxide and nitric oxide and their reaction products regulate many processes, such as control of vascular tone and thus blood pressure. They also play a key role in the intermediary metabolism of various biological compounds.

In biology

Because of their reactivity, excessive amounts of these free radicals can lead to cell injury.

In the body, they attack the cell membrane, protein molecules, etc., and the cell nucleus. They cause aging and may also contribute too many diseases such as cancer, stroke, myocardial infarction, diabetes and major disorders. Many forms of cancer are thought to be the result of reactions between free radicals and DNA, potentially resulting in mutations that can adversely affect the cell cycle and potentially lead to malignancy. Some of the symptoms of aging such as atherosclerosis are also attributed to free-radical induced oxidation of cholesterol to 7-ketocholesterol. In addition, free radicals contribute to alcohol-induced liver damage, perhaps more than alcohol itself. Free radicals produced by cigarette smoke are implicated in inactivation of alpha 1-antitrypsin in the lung. This process promotes the development of emphysema.

*"Free radicals may also be involved in Parkinson's disease, senile and drug-induced deafness, schizophrenia, and Alzheimer's. The classic free-radical syndrome, the iron-storage disease hemochromatosis, is typically associated with a constellation of free-radical-related symptoms including movement disorder, psychosis, skin pigmentary melanin abnormalities, deafness, arthritis, and diabetes mellitus. The free-radical theory of aging proposes that free radicals underlie the aging process itself."*

**Source:** https://www.news-medical.net/life-sciences/What-is-Metabolism.aspx

The two most important oxygen-centered free radicals are superoxide and hydroxyl radical. They derive from molecular oxygen under reducing conditions.

Reactive oxygen species (ROS) are species such as superoxide, hydrogen peroxide, and hydroxyl radical, commonly associated with cell damage. ROS is formed as a natural by-product of the normal metabolism of oxygen and have important roles in cell signaling. Oxybenzone has been found to form free radicals in sunlight and therefore may be associated with cell damage. This only occurred when it was combined with other ingredients commonly found in sunscreens, like titanium oxide and octyl methoxycinnamate.

ROS attack the polyunsaturated fatty acid, linoleic acid, to form a series of 13-Hydroxyoctadecadienoic acid and 9-Hydroxyoctadecadienoic acid products that serve as signaling molecules that may trigger responses that counter the tissue injury, which caused their formation. ROS attacks other polyunsaturated fatty acids, e.g. arachidonic acid and docosahexaenoic acid.

\*\*\*\*\*\*

The body has a number of mechanisms to minimize free-radical-induced damage and to repair the damage that occurs, such as the enzymes superoxide dismutase, catalase, glutathione peroxidase and glutathione reeducates.

In addition, antioxidants play a key role in these defense mechanisms. These are often the three vitamins, vitamin A, vitamin C and vitamin E and polyphenol antioxidants. Furthermore, there is good evidence indicating that bilirubin and uric acid can act as antioxidants to help neutralize certain free radicals.

# Protein synthesis in cell

Protein synthesis is the process whereby biological cells generate new proteins. It is balanced by the loss of cellular proteins, is regulated at multiple steps. They Include two processes: (source: https://en.wikipedia.org/wiki/Protein_biosynthesis )

- Transcription (phenomena of RNA synthesis from DNA template):

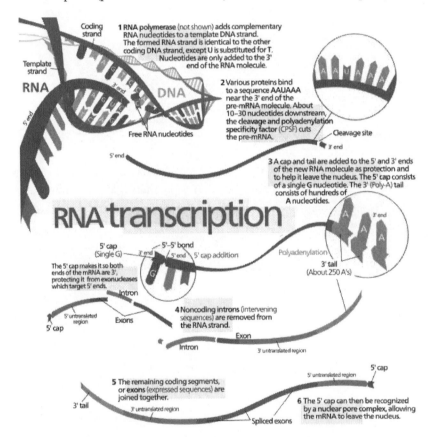

- Translation (phenomena of the amino acid assembly from RNA):

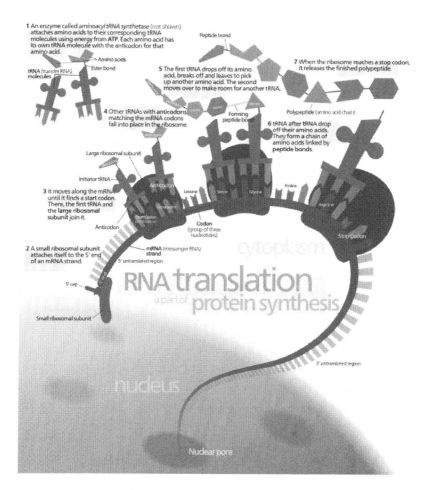

1 An enzyme called *aminoacyl tRNA synthetase* (not shown) attaches amino acids to their corresponding tRNA molecules using energy from ATP. Each amino acid has its own tRNA molecule with the anticodon for that amino acid.

Peptide bond

Amino acids

tRNA (transfer RNA) molecules

Ester bond

5 The first tRNA drops off its amino acid, breaks off and leaves to pick up another amino acid. The second moves over to make room for another tRNA.

7 When the ribosome reaches a stop codon, it releases the finished polypeptide.

4 Other tRNAs with anticodons matching the mRNA codons fall into place in the ribosome.

Forming peptide bond

Polypeptide (amino acid chain)

6 tRNA after tRNA drop off their amino acids. They form a chain of amino acids linked by peptide bonds.

Large ribosomal subunit

Initiator tRNA

3 It moves along the mRNA until it finds a start codon. There, the first tRNA and the large ribosomal subunit join it.

Anticodon

Leucine

Serine

Glycine

Proline

Arginine

Anticodon

Codon (group of three nucleotides)

Stop codon

2 A small ribosomal subunit attaches itself to the 5' end of an mRNA strand.

mRNA (messenger RNA) strand

5' untranslated region

5' cap

cytoplasm

RNA translation

a part of protein synthesis

Small ribosomal subunit

3' untranslated region

nucleus

Nuclear pore

RNA is transcribed in the nucleus; it is transported to the cytoplasm and translated by the ribosome.

Translation is an essential part of the biosynthetic pathway, with the generation of messenger RNA (mRNA), aminoacylation of transfer RNA (tRNA).

The cistron DNA is transcribed into the RNA is used as a template for synthesis of a polypeptide chain. Protein will often be synthesized directly by translating mRNA.

In protein synthesis, a succession of tRNA molecules charged with appropriate amino acids are brought together with a mRNA molecule and matched up through the anti-codons of the tRNA with successive codons of the mRNA. The amino acids are then linked together to extend the growing protein chain, and the tRNAs, no longer carrying amino acids, are released. *"This whole complex of processes is carried out by the ribosome, formed of two main chains of RNA, called ribosomal RNA (rRNA), and more than 50 different proteins."*

**Source:** https://en.wikipedia.org/wiki/Protein_biosynthesis

Transcription, RNA synthesis from DNA template. In transcription, an mRNA chain is generated, with one strand of the DNA double helix in the genome as a template. Transcription occurs in the cell nucleus, where the DNA is held. The general RNA structure is very similar to the DNA structure. The single strand of mRNA leaves the nucleus through nuclear pores and migrates into the cytoplasm.

Translation: The synthesis of proteins from RNA is known as translation. In eukaryotes, translation occurs in the cytoplasm, where the ribosomes are located. Ribosomes are made of a small and large subunit that surrounds the mRNA.

In translation, messenger RNA (mRNA) is decoded to produce a specific polypeptide. This uses an mRNA sequence as a template to guide the synthesis of a chain of amino acids that form a protein.

In activation, the correct amino acid (AA) is joined to the correct transfer RNA (tRNA). Initiation, involves the small subunit of the ribosome, binding to 5' end of mRNA with the help of initiation factors (IF). Elongation occurs when the next aminoacyl-tRNA (charged tRNA) in line binds to the ribosome. Termination of the polypeptide happens when the A site of the ribosome faces a stop codon. When this happens, no tRNA can recognize it, but releasing factor can recognize nonsense codons and causes the release of the polypeptide chain.

# PART III: WIN THE FIGHT AGAINST CANCER AGAIN

### Drink the water of ten coconuts; melanoma was "kicked out"

Melanoma is the most dangerous form of skin cancer. Cancer cells grow when the DNA of a skin cell is mutated, often caused by ultraviolet radiation from the sun, forming malignant tumors. These tumors originate from melanocyte cells that produce pigment in the floor of the epidermis. Melanoma is usually like a mole. Some develop from a mole. Most melanomas are black or brown, but may also be in different colors:

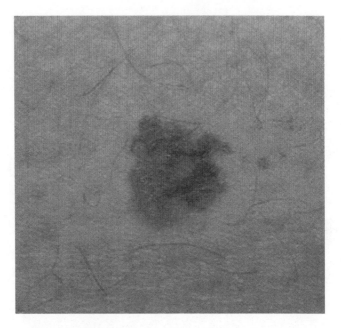

Melanoma annually kills more 10,000 people in the United States alone. If melanoma is detected early, the disease can be treated. Conversely, if the disease has progressed to a late stage and metastasis to other parts of the body, treatment is difficult and mortality is high. Although this disease is not the most common form of skin cancer, it is responsible for most deaths.

As I wrote, 4 years ago, the mole under my left eye suddenly itched and grew; I thought it would turn into melanoma. I applied the diet with the theoretical basis being that cutting off source animal protein in the diet would mean that the tumors have no material to grow and would die. More positive, I was not only fasting but also not any thing eat,I only drunk coconut juice for about 10 days, by the end of which mole had fallen out.

Thus, the mole is transformed into malignant tumors, so it is affected by the diet. This suggests that the theory of cancer treatment with vegetarian diets is correct.

Let me remind you a story at the beginning of this book. I have a friend who has liver cancer because he has been infected with the B virus for a long time. He has surgery in Cho Ray hospital. I advised him to be a strict vegetarian and if possible, not to eat anything during the time that he can tolerate. As a result, when he went back to the clinic after three months of surgery, the doctor found no recurrence of the tumor. When the liver has four such tumors, doctors cannot completely take the cancer cells off the liver. So, after 3 months, my friend has been a vegetarian, there has not been any tumor growth reported. The theory of using vegetarian food has again been proven.

\*\*\*\*\*\*

And even to these days, the theory of using vegetarian food to fight cancer has been proven more than once.

As I wrote at the beginning of this book, one day I came to the bank to withdraw some money for consumption. I took the order number and waited a little while. I watched the clock and startled, I saw my wrist, the place I wear my watch, had a purple-black spot! Sadly! Because I knew it was definitely a melanoma! Although I had been successful in treating melanoma, I was still very depressed. If this time I'm not successful what will happen? The method drawn from using food to fight cancer is thought to be very simple, but difficult to implement. If we don't eat anything, we are faced with extreme hunger. It is terrible to suffer from hunger and try to overcome it. But between hunger and death, one must choose one. And I chose hunger.

The work was completed, from the bank I went home. It was a weekend, I saw my wife cooking in a large pot "Bun Bo Hue". The smell of food spread everywhere. I am hungry, how can I not eat? I told my wife:

- Today I will eat normally once again; tomorrow I will resume "hunger strike" again!

My wife was surprised:

- What happened?

I did not want my wife to worry; I hide the truth and replied:

- Only to lose weight!

At lunch, I ate deliciously together with my wife and children "Bun Bo Hue". Drunk a few cans of Heineken beer for the happy life. Ate as if I will never eat "Bun Bo Hue" again!

\*\*\*\*\*\*

The next morning, I went to the market to buy ten coconuts, it cost me $5 only in the US money. I drained water from 10 coconuts and stored in the refrigerator to drink for two days.

It's great! Only after two days, I noticed the purple-black spot had changed a lot:

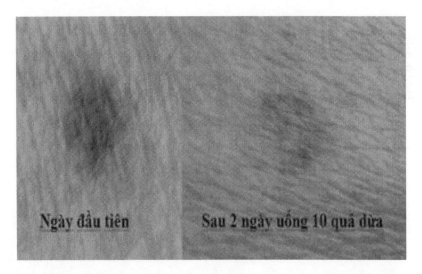

Ngày đầu tiên          Sau 2 ngày uống 10 quả dừa

And this time, I only drunk coconut water in those two days. I don't want to be cured early because I wanted to try eating other vegetarian foods to see the purple-black spot, how it was changing.

The next days I only ate soup made from beetroot, carrots, potatoes, and white radish. I only ate vegetables and tubers. And finally, after about 10 days, once again, I had won the fight against skin cancer! The purple-black spot had completely disappeared!

Interestingly, since melanoma is on the skin, we can see the effect of diet on it easily.

The picture I took of my own wrist shown below shows the melanoma gradually being completely destroyed by the diet that cuts off animal protein completely:

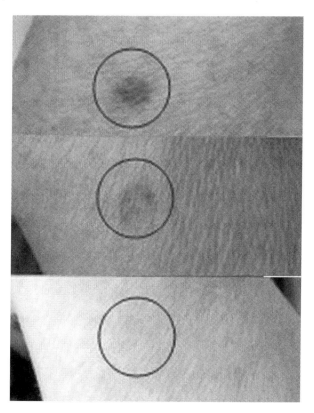

## DISCUSSION

The human body synthesizes many amino acids, it just does not synthesize the essential amino acids. So they need to be provided from what we eat. In fact, the body needs to provide little protein for its activities. The lifespan of each type of tissue depends upon the workload endured by its cells.

There are cells that live for a very long time. Lymphocytes: 2 months - a year (highly variable). Red blood cells: 4 months. Macrophages: months - years. Endothelial cells: months - years. Pancreas cells: 1 year or more. Bone cells: 25 - 30 years. An adult human liver cell replaces itself about once every year to one year and a half. The entire human skeleton cells are thought to be replaced every 10 years or so in adults. Therefore, the amount of protein in meals often exceeds the body's protein requirements.

This has been proven by many people who eat only brown rice and sesame salt, not only live a normal life but also a healthy one, meaning their body is not lacking in protein. In converse, if we eat too much protein daily, it not only harm the body but also just "fatten" the cancer tumors. So, we can confirm, also as we eat too many carbohydrates, it causes diabetes, eating too much animal fat and cholesterol causes cardiovascular disease, eating excess protein can also cause cancer.

So to fight cancer, we need to do the opposite, as in the old battles, people often cut out the enemy's way of transporting food.

Only simply thus which not everyone understands, and when people understand that thing, not everyone can do it right .

Los Angeles

2-9-2017

ĐÔNG LA

# APPENDIX

The story about a "Holy Lady" which has strange ability to cure cancer

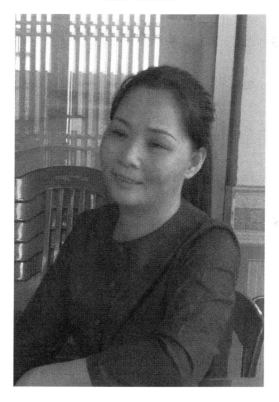

*(Ms. Vu Thi Hoa)*

On the VTV1 (channel 1 of Vietnam Television), 20-10-2013, the program "Return from memory" No. 22 shocked the public. Female journalist THU

UYEN talked about two women: Phan Thi Bich Hang and Vu Thi Hoa that they are fraud "take advantage of the bones and blood of the fallen heroes". These two women are two of those who can communicate with the soul of the dead in Vietnam. They went and helped to find the missing bones of fallen heroes. As a writer, I read a lot and I clearly know them. So I know for sure that they are not phishing but just Journalist. Thu Uyen lied about them.

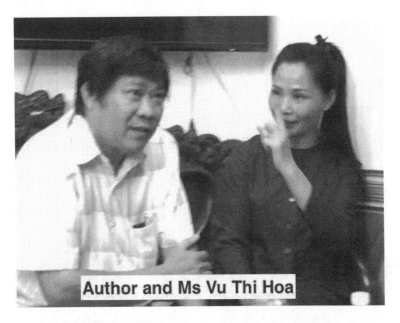

**Author and Ms Vu Thi Hoa**

On October 26, 2013, I wrote a post on my blog "A philanthropical program but inhuman!" to protect those two women. Colonel Dao Van Su, former correspondent of "People's Army," an acquaintance of Ms. Vu Thi Hoa, wrote that I am a brave writer, have defended the innocent which he didn't dare to do. So, I started getting used to a woman with strange abilities that I never saw. Then Ms. Vu Thi Hoa and I met many times, developing close bonds like relatives. I witnessed so many of her strange abilities such as communicating with the soul of the dead, looking through space and time, looking deep underground, etc. and she could also cure cancer.

Today I just wrote a few things, eg. she in Hanoi saw me doing something in Saigon and she can also see my son in the US!

One time she said that under a family's bedroom in Hoc Mon district, more than 100 years ago, a girl was buried, so the family had many bad t omens. Eg. as the eldest son had an accident; his brothers hold the knife to fight each other, etc.

She helped that family get the girl's bones up, but having been buried for so long underneath there, they could only find mud and a small plate buried with the girl. I did not sleep all night to see some people dig up a whole 2 .7 m deep at the foot of the wall to get some mud and, strangely, there was a small plate which Ms. Hoa described earlier.

Another time, I also witnessed the digging deep of 1.7 m, also under the wall of a house to take up a set of bones of a fallen heroes. Mrs. Hoa said first, only has rested a few pieces of bones, pieces of clothing, and special, there are a gold-coated tooth and a plastic pen. Then, all as she said!

I took a lot of pictures of people who have been helped by Ms. Hoa. She helps them with spiritual issues and healing. They knelt in front of her; admired her as before a Bodhisattva:

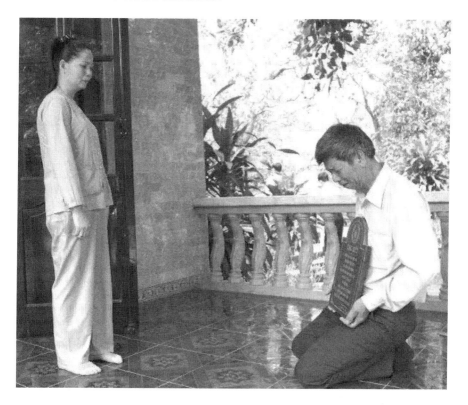

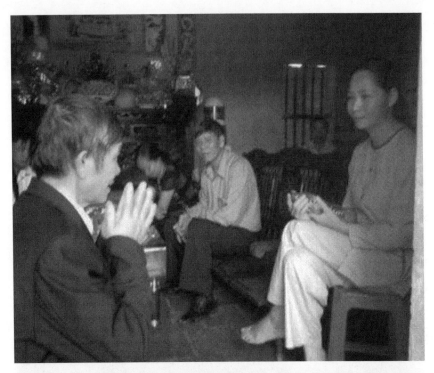

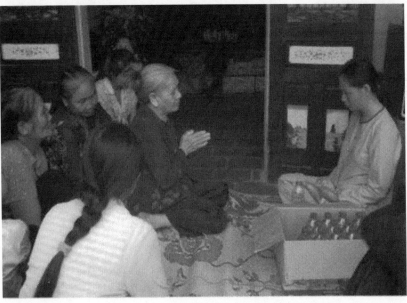

***

For healing, she often gave his patients coconut water and bottled water to drink after she has "transmitted energy". She only holds in her hands the bottles of water at normal temperature, it could be hot at 80-900 C. People who took that water often said that she was "Gia hộ" for them, as was blessed, received the "holy water".

She also often to give patients use the Medicinal plants in the forest, at most is one species root of tree that was not present in any prescription of Oriental medicine and used her mystical energy to heal. About the ability to cure cancer of Ms. Vu Thi Hoa, I am only going to discuss two examples.

1-The first was Ms. Chu Thi Xoan, who had a brain tumor.

This is the content of the letter to Ms. Vu Thi Hoa:

"Dear Ms. Vu Thi Hoa, like my mother!

My name is Chu Thi Xoan,

Hamlet 14, village Đanh Xá, District Kim Bảng, provincial Hà Nam, Identity card number issued by Ha Nam police: 168471375.

Now, I same as a person come back from the place of death, I would like to express gratitude, thank you saved me alive.

I have brain cancer: I have brain cancer:

**BỆNH VIỆN K**
**KHOA CHẨN ĐOÁN HÌNH ẢNH**
Tel: 9.365.823; 0913.505.906

# GIẤY CHỤP CỘNG HƯỞNG TỪ
## (MRI)

MRI scan paper

**Họ và tên**: CHU THỊ XOAN        **Tuổi**: 52        Nữ

**Khoa**: PK — Bs Hảo

**Chẩn đoán làm sàng**: U màng não

**Yêu cầu MRI**:        Sọ não.

## KỸ THUẬT:

Chụp cộng hưởng từ sọ não với các chuỗi xung T1W, T2W, FLAR, COR T1 theo các mặt phẳng ngang, đứng dọc, đứng ngang không và có tiêm thuốc đối quang từ.

## KẾT QUẢ:

- Không thấy tổn thương hay khối choán chỗ trong não vùng trên và dưới lều. Nhồi máu cũ vùng nhân xám sừng trước não thất bên 2 bên.
- Hệ thống não thất không giãn, cân đối, dịch não tuỷ có tín hiệu đồng nhất.
- Đường giữa không bị di lệch.
- Không thấy bất thường ở giao thoa thị giác và các dây thần kinh sọ.
- Tuyến yên có kích thước và tín hiệu bình thường. Cuống tuyến yên thanh mảnh, cân đối.
- Không có viêm xoang khối mặt và sau.
- Mắt : nhãn cầu và hậu nhãn cầu bình thường.
- Vùng vòm hai bên và sau không dầy .

*Kết luận*: Không xác định U não- nhồi máu cũ vùng sừng nhân xám sắt não thất bên 2 bên □ Không có viêm xoang khối mặt và xoang sau □ Không dầy thành vòm 2 bên và sau .

Ngày 15 tháng 1 năm 2013

Bác sỹ chuyên khoa

BS. NGUYỄN ĐĂNG HÀ

# ĐƠN THUỐC

Họ tên:.....*Chu......Thi......Xoan*....................Tuổi:...*5 2*

Địa chỉ :....................*Hà....Nam*...........................................

Căn bệnh:............*U....não....Thất....bên....+ IV*

1/ *Tôn hợp TK 30  x   46*

*ngày uống HU chia 2 lần*

*sau ăn*

2/ *Dexamethazon 0,5 mg x  20c*

*ngày uống 2U chia 2 lần*

Ngày.*16*.tháng.*2*....năm.*2012*

**Y.Bác sĩ**

Họ tên:...*BS Vũ Ngọc Liên*

G 016 VD-11

It has tormented me for a long time. I have been treated in hospitals. Doctors told me to go home to wait for death. That was on February 15, 2012. Go home, I was tortured by the pain, my brain is like broken. I have to hit my head on the wall so that the pain outside can reduce the pain inside.

On 16/2/2012, I was lucky to meet you. You looked at me as the child with compassionate eyes of The Bodhisattva. You gave me three coconuts; I was drinking the water of coconut one by one:

Drunk first fruit: the pain reduced.

Drunk the second fruit: the pain reduced even further.

Drunk Third fruit:

The pain was subsiding gradually as if it was the work of magic! I don't know what to say to show gratitude, I can only say "thousand times thank you!"

Dear mother!

You are like my Mother, I was born again. With me, you are the Bodhisattva Avalokiteshvara descending to earth to save humanity. Only the Buddha can save me carefree without receiving any money from my family.

On January 15, 2013, I went to the hospital again, doctors concluded that I no longer had cancer. I have returned to normal life and went to work as before.

A mother's child

Chu Thi Xoan

**Thư cảm ơn**

Kính gửi Cô Vũ Thị **Thank you letter**

Con là: Chu Thị Xoan

Địa chỉ: Xóm 14, thôn Danh Xá, xã Ngọc Sơn, huyện Kim Bảng, tỉnh Hà Nam

CMTND số: 168471375 do Công an tỉnh Hà Nam cấp.

Con viết thư này xin bày tỏ lòng tri ân của người từ cõi chết trở về xin ngàn lần cảm ơn Cô cùng các phật tử của Cô đã cứu con sống lại.

Con nhớ như in những việc làm tâm đức của Cô đã cứu con thoát khỏi bệnh ung thư não – Căn bệnh quái ác đã hành hạ con. Con đã đi chữa trị khắp các bệnh viện, bác sỹ đều bó tay và trả con về với gia đình để chờ chết, giấy tờ bệnh viện con vẫn còn giữ nguyên, đó là ngày 15/2/2012. Con được gia đình đưa từ bệnh viện về nhà với những cơn đau hành hạ tưởng như vỡ óc, con liên tiếp đập đầu vào tường để lấy cơn đau ở ngoài làm giảm cơn đau bên trong. Cả gia đình con lo lắng ngồi nhìn con chờ chết mà không có cách nào giúp con được. Ngày 16/2/2012 con được gặp Cô, cô nhìn con với ánh mắt thương cảm, Cô có tâm từ bi của Phật bà Quan thế âm Bồ Tát giang tay cứu nhân độ thế, Cô nhận lời chữa bệnh cho con. Cô ban cho con 3 quả dứa, con uống từng quả:

Quả thứ nhất: Trong người con như nhẹ hẳn, cơn đau bớt xuống.

Quả thứ hai: Cơn đau đớn thưa dần

Quả thứ ba: Những cơn đau không còn liên tục như trước nữa. Như một phép nhiệm màu Cô ạ, phúc đức nhà con được gặp Cô, con không biết nói gì để tỏ lòng biết ơn, con chỉ biết ngàn lần đội ơn Cô mà thôi. Sau đó vài hôm Cô cho các phật tử lấy thuốc nam cho con uống, những củ thuốc nam mà Cô ban cho con là do các phật tử của Cô phải đào sâu dưới lòng đất, đi tìm trong rừng già xa thẳm. Con biết sự vất vả đó mà không biết nói gì hơn ngoài lời cảm ơn sâu sắc.

Cô ơi, Cô đã một lần nữa sinh ra con, Cô cứu con từ cõi chết trở về, với con Cô là Phật bà Quan thế âm Bồ Tát giáng trần cứu nhân độ thế. Cô cứu con thoát bệnh hiểm nghèo mà không hề nhận một đồng tiền nào của con và gia đình. Ngày 15/1/2013 con đã đi bệnh viện khám lại, bác sỹ kết luận con không có bệnh gì. Con đã trở lại cuộc sống bình thường và đã đi làm trở lại như trước đây.

Phúc đức của cô ban đại gia đình con đã được hưởng. Cô là đại ân nhân của con và toàn thể gia đình. Gia đình con một lần nữa xin tỏ lòng biết ơn Cô và xin khắc cốt ghi tâm những ân đức mà Cô trao cho chúng con.

*Chu thị Xoan*

*Xoan*

Thưa nhà văn Đông La!

Tôi là Chu Thị Xoan, bệnh nhân của ung thư não đã được Cô Vũ Thị Hòa chữa khỏi. Qua trang blog của anh, tôi đã được đọc những bài viết chính luận, những bài viết về cô Vũ Thị Hòa tôi thấy rất ngưỡng mộ và khâm phục anh. Tôi có tâm nguyện muốn xin nhờ anh đăng giúp lời cảm ơn của tôi tới đại ân nhân của tôi tới Cô Vũ Thị Hòa và các phật tử của Cô. Để tỏ lòng biết ơn sâu sắc của tôi tới Cô – Người đã giúp tôi thoát khỏi lưỡi hái tử thần.

*Chu thị Xoan*

*Xoan*

2- second is Ms. Trương Thị Ngọc Minh:

This woman lives in Vung Tau (phone number: 0919.318.479).

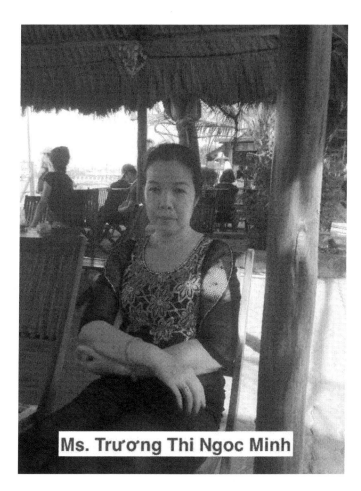

Ms. Trương Thi Ngoc Minh

In 2009, when she went to the hospital, she was shocked by the doctor's diagnosis that she had stage 2-bladder cancer. That year, she had surgery twice and had chemotherapy to prevent metastasis.

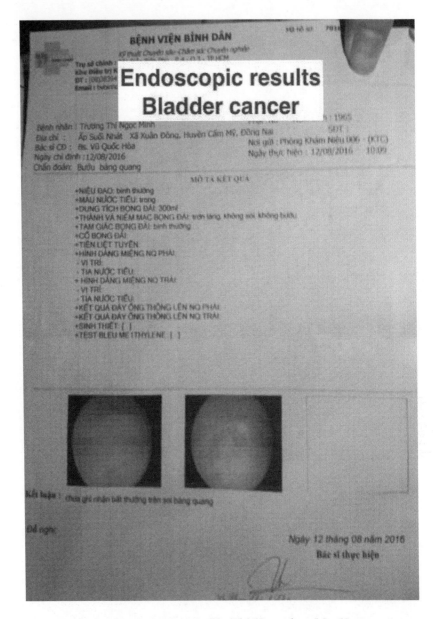

**Endoscopic results Bladder cancer**

BỆNH VIỆN BÌNH DÂN

Bệnh nhân : Trương Thị Ngọc Minh
Địa chỉ : Ấp Suối Nhất, Xã Xuân Đông, Huyện Cẩm Mỹ, Đồng Nai
Bác sĩ CĐ : Bs. Vũ Quốc Hòa
Ngày chỉ định : 12/08/2016
Chẩn đoán: Bướu bàng quang

Nơi giữ : Phòng Khám Niệu 006 - (KTC)
Ngày thực hiện : 12/08/2016

MÔ TẢ KẾT QUẢ

+NIỆU ĐẠO: bình thường
+MÀU NƯỚC TIỂU: trong
+DUNG TÍCH BỌNG ĐÁI: 300ml
+THÀNH VÀ NIÊM MẠC BỌNG ĐÁI: trơn láng, không sỏi, không bướu
+TAM GIÁC BỌNG ĐÁI: bình thường
+CỔ BỌNG ĐÁI:
+TIỀN LIỆT TUYẾN:
+HÌNH DẠNG MIỆNG NQ PHẢI:
  - VỊ TRÍ:
  - TIA NƯỚC TIỂU:
+ HÌNH DẠNG MIỆNG NQ TRÁI:
  - VỊ TRÍ:
  - TIA NƯỚC TIỂU:
+KẾT QUẢ ĐẨY ỐNG THÔNG LÊN NQ PHẢI:
+KẾT QUẢ ĐẨY ỐNG THÔNG LÊN NQ TRÁI:
+SINH THIẾT [ ]
+TEST BLEU MÉTHYLÈNE [ ]

Kết luận : chưa ghi nhận bất thường trên soi bàng quang

Đề nghị:

Ngày 12 tháng 08 năm 2016
Bác sĩ thực hiện

In August 2011, Ms. Minh met Ms. Vu Thi Hoa when Ms. Hoa went to help find the missing bones of fallen heroes in May Tau commune, Xuyen Moc district, Dong Nai province.

Ms. Hoa looked at Minh's haggard body and said, "I will cure you of this disease with my medication. It is important that you believe and cooks medicines to drink regularly ... ". Ms. Minh is very happy. She did exactly what Ms. Hoa said to her and had a very unexpected result.

She feels her health gradually improve. After 4 months of taking medicine of Ms. Hoa, Ms. Minh went to Binh Dan Hospital (Ho Chi Minh City). The doctor examined her and said she was cured.

By September 2015, Ms. Minh was once again in panic because of the recurrence of bladder cancer. After examination at Binh Dan hospital, doctors said she had to undergo surgery, radiation therapy because it has metastasized.

At that time, Ms. Hoa was in Sai Gon City. With the ability to see from far, Ms. Hoa knew Ms. Minh had cancer recurrence. She called Ms. Minh to meet her right away. Then within 4 months, Ms. Minh arrived at Ms. Hoa's place for treatment. In early 2016; she came home in a happy mood. Because on August 12/2016, she went to see her doctor again, the doctor confirmed she had been cured after examining her!

\*\*\*\*\*\*

These stories about Ms. Vu Thi Hoa are more like myths but it is the truth. I used to be a researcher of pharmaceutical chemistry, at the same time; I am also a Writer, critic, so I'm not superstitious. I just want to say that life has a lot of mysterious things out of sight of modern science. Just like modern medicine, many still do not believe that the vegetarian diet can cure cancer, but it is still true.

*Los Angeles*

*2-9-2017*

*ĐÔNG LA*

65893676R00050

Made in the USA
Middletown, DE
05 March 2018